"A powerful analysis of the current a   ue the yoga industry due to colonization and   *nce* is a transformative book that can reorient the Western yoga industry by bringing attention and care to South Asian, Indian, BIPOC, Desi and queer voices and experiences, while at the same time challenging colonization, white supremacy, cultural appropriation and other systems of oppression.

Graham's book is accessible and clear, offering readers an opportunity to learn and do better. She links the benefit of the practice with clarity to the powerful work of social change. Her direct approach invites self-reflection, compassion and care. She gives us delightful 'practice breaks' throughout that invite integration of this important work. This book is a must-read for yoga studios, training schools, teachers and practitioners."

Susanna Barkataki, author of *Embrace Yoga's Roots*

"Many of us dedicated to the liberatory path of Yoga know and understand the challenge of engaging with such a profound path that has for some time been disrupted by colonization, capitalism and white supremacy. In a clear, direct and compassionate voice enriched by years of authentic practice, Dr Stacie C.C. Graham opens up a way forward for practitioners, teachers and yoga communities to do the real work of decentring the violence of exclusivity and recentring the profound and accessible liberatory teachings. *Yoga as Resistance* will become an important guidebook helping all of us to reconnect to the real expression of Yoga."

Lama Rod Owens, author of *Love and Rage:*
The Path of Liberation through Anger

"This is an important book for our times. Structural racism, inequity and inequality are rife throughout societies – and yoga is no different. There has been a systems-level exclusion of people of colour, and anyone else whose face or body shape was deemed not to fit. Far from the unity and oneness expressed in Patanjali, we have had far too much yoga that is obsessed with gymnastic shapes (usually slim white women) and has insulted the cultural and wisdom heritage of the Yoga tradition in favour of a mindset reminiscent of colonial appropriation. Yoga's reaction to all of this has been a predictable mix of guilt and denial – there is no problem; me, racist? *Yoga as Resistance* is a wake-up call to the un-awakened, providing the information and analysis to become fully conscious of structures of inequity and exclusion in yoga and the importance of dismantling them. Dr Graham leads the reader step by step through the conceptual framework and vocabulary needed to address these issues, alongside practical strategies for studios, teacher training schools and yoga brand holders to change direction. All this important work is lightened by insights from yogic texts, journaling prompts and practices to enable the reader to reflect and embed the knowledge to become agents of change.

For many of us, yoga on and off the mat has always been a foundation for the struggle for social justice, equity, equality and inclusion. Yoga is about health, wellness, and transformation. It should also be Yoga as resistance."

Paul Fox, Chief Operating Officer of the Yoga In Healthcare Alliance and former Chair of the British Wheel of Yoga

"Through the lens of social justice activism, Dr Stacie Graham shares information, light bulb moments, 'unlearning tips', yoga practices, journaling prompts and real-life examples to invite yoga studio owners, yoga schools, yoga teachers and yoga practitioners to think about and reflect on how yoga is taught, who teaches it, and who practises it within their locations. She challenges us to engage in self-study – *syādhyāya* – and to distinguish our own personal truth from the Truth – *satya* – and to face our own hypocrisy when we claim that yoga means unity, all appearances to the contrary. But that's not all. She tells us how to make the changes within our business practices, our yoga schools, our yoga studios and ourselves that will demonstrate the diversity, equity and inclusion that we advocate, so that these are more than just words on a page. If you want to make a difference, if you want to be part of real change, this is an important read."

Gail Parker, Ph.D., E-RYT 500, C-IAYT, psychologist, yoga therapist educator, President of the Black Yoga Teachers Alliance Board of Directors, and author of *Restorative Yoga for Ethnic and Race-Based Stress and Trauma* and *Transforming Ethnic and Race-Based Traumatic Stress With Yoga*

"*Yoga as Resistance* is a voice of compassionate strength. Dr Graham's writing empowers her readers to see yoga as a tool that can translate our inner experience into an outer form of social justice and change. Inspiring, challenging and forgiving, *Yoga as Resistance* confirms why racial equity and justice sit unmistakably within the framework of classical yoga philosophies. By grounding theory into tangible practices and action, she brings ancient teachings into clear, present-day relief. I hope her book will be read far and wide by people within the yoga community and serve to move our individual and collective experiences together towards greater equality, liberation and freedom."

**Mimi Kuo-Deemer, author and teacher of
meditation and the movement arts**

"*Yoga as Resistance* is a call to action that artfully explores a much-needed pathway towards a more equitable and sustainable yoga and wellness industry. Dr Graham offers an accessible, engaging and practical guide that draws on relatable stories while balancing self-enquiry and equitable strategies. Highly recommended to all sincere students, teachers and studios as a go-to resource for driving change on both an individual and collective level. As Dr Graham states, the smallest well-informed actions will pave the way for lasting change; this book asks us all to act, meaningfully and intentionally, and offers doable steps and refined tools to aid us all in the process."

Julia Midland, Founder and Director of The OmPowerment Project

"Dr Graham has given us a gift in writing this book and offering specific, step-by-step guidance for anyone in the yoga industry to make their work more just and equitable. *Yoga as Resistance* offers a clear call to yoga teachers, studios and brands to do the often-difficult work of examining our motivations, assumptions and practices. It also outlines a pathway of accountability and action that we all must take in order for our work to have integrity and align with the true spirit of Yoga which is resisting the status quo and guiding people towards liberation personally and collectively."

**Hala Khouri, M.A, SEP, E-RYT, co-founder of Off the Mat,
Into the World and trainer for Collective Resilience Yoga**

"This book is a call to action – to go beyond poses and performance and live Yoga out in the world. Through Stacie's guidance, we return to the wisdom tradition and recalibrate to the practice of justice that is inherent to Yoga. It is a tool and a journey towards the freedom we are yearning for."

Kerri Kelly, author of *American Detox: The Myth of Wellness and How We Can Truly Heal*

"Wise, fierce and compassionate, Dr Stacie C.C. Graham calls us into action to practice deeply and do the work for real change. *Yoga As Resistance* offers a clear framework to create equity and inclusion, transform ideas into action, and break free from oppressive dominant culture in the yoga and wellness industry. As a white woman and teacher of yoga, this book offers essential ways to dig deep, listen on every level, identify blocks that prevent showing up to do the work, face the fears of 'getting it wrong', and rise up to create yoga spaces that benefit all. *Yoga As Resistance* is an essential resource for every yoga teacher, and I feel it should be in the core curriculum of every yoga teacher training."

Sianna Sherman, she/her, visionary of the Rasa Yoga Collective

ABOUT THE AUTHOR

Dr Stacie C.C. Graham is a sought-after expert on leadership, equity and inclusion. She works internationally as an executive coach, management and strategy consultant. She has been published and her work featured in several publications, including for the BBC, *Essence*, *Forbes*, *gal-dem*, the *Guardian* and *USA Today*.

Graham is the founder of OYA: Body–Mind–Spirit Retreats, which is a holistic wellness brand dedicated to improving the mental, physical and emotional health of Black women and women of colour by making holistic wellness practices more accessible. It was the first such brand to explicitly work with these communities in the United Kingdom. OYA Retreats deliver holistic movement and mindfulness experiences and workshop immersions with community members across Europe, North America and Africa.

Graham holds a master's degree in economics from Ruprecht-Karls University and a doctoral degree in psychology from the University of Osnabrück. She is registered with Yoga Alliance as an experienced Haṭha Yoga teacher (E-RYT 500) and is a certified mindfulness teacher.

YOGA AS RESISTANCE

YOGA AS RESISTANCE

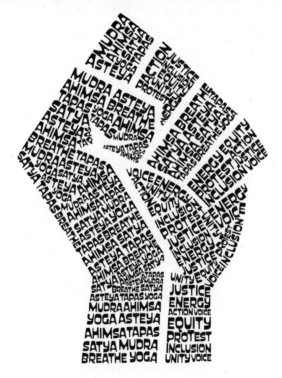

EQUITY AND INCLUSION ON AND OFF THE MAT

Dr Stacie C.C. Graham

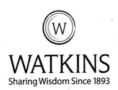

WATKINS

Sharing Wisdom Since 1893

This edition first published in the UK and USA in 2022 by
Watkins, an imprint of Watkins Media Limited
Unit 11, Shepperton House
89-93 Shepperton Road
London
N1 3DF

enquiries@watkinspublishing.com

1 3 5 7 9 10 8 6 4 2

Designed and Typeset by Lapiz

Printed and bound in the United Kingdom by TJ Books Ltd

A CIP record for this book is available from the British Library

ISBN: 978-1-78678-640-1 (Paperback)
ISBN: 978-1-78678-641-8 (eBook)

www.watkinspublishing.com

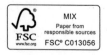

MIX
Paper from
responsible sources
FSC® C013056
www.fsc.org

For Guruji, all my teachers and the teacher within.

ACKNOWLEDGEMENTS

This book represents a culmination of personal work that began decades ago. I bow deeply to the ancestors and elders who came before me and whose collective wisdom resides within me. I offer gratitude to the activists, artists and teachers who have worked tirelessly for our collective freedom. To the unsung heroines, whose stories we may never know.

To my mother, Mattie Burden, who prepared me for the challenges of life in a short amount of time. She was a woman of faith who practised compassion and empathy. And she had an exceptional amount of patience for my inquisitiveness concerning race matters.

To Oliver Stahnke and Little Hunter Pumpkin, I thank you for offering the space I needed while I was working at capacity while writing this book and still fulfilling other obligations. Thank you for listening, for offering encouraging words to keep me going, and generally making it possible for me to travel the world and follow this path.

I'm grateful to Danny Brose for encouraging me to give yoga a try. Without that push, I would not have set off on this journey, at least not so early. I bow to all of my Yoga and mindfulness teachers with whom I have had the pleasure to study, directly and through their published teachings. There are many; however, I would like to mention Sue Darling Elivique who always found time to teach more than āsana and often connected the practice to the three guṇas. As a teacher, she demonstrates what is possible no matter the studio environment or length of class.

I'm grateful to Dr Suresh Nampuri for the endless emotional support while I was writing my doctoral dissertation, the gentle yet firm nudge to take a break, and the much-needed support as I travelled through India for the first time. To Mansi Sehgal and Prerna Lulla for welcoming me to Mumbai with such kindness and joy. To Hema Nagpal for building and maintaining a friendship. Your generosity is unmatched: hosting me in Mumbai, spending time with me in Washington DC, helping me discover the teacher training that I was genuinely looking for, and cheering me on as I founded my own wellness space. Thank you.

To all of my students, teacher trainees, clients, workshop participants and OYA community members, I would like to express my sincere gratitude. We create learning environments together. I was able to write this book because of the work that we did and continue to do – together. Thank you for showing up, trying your best, and committing to the ongoing work.

A special thanks to the women who opened their hearts and shared their truth for this book: Aya-Nikole Cook of Haji Healing Salon, Elisa Shankle of HealHaus, and Twanna Doherty of Yogamatters. Your words are so magnificent and beautiful and perfectly encapsulate what is possible in collectively created spaces. Deep gratitude to Aya and Elisa for the healing spaces you provide to your communities with authenticity, care and love.

To Anya Hayes, who believed in this book from the very first moment hearing of it. Thank you for all of your support. To Fiona Robertson for picking up the baton and carrying it over the finish line. Thank you to all of the Watkins Publishing team for believing in the book and its author.

Finally, I am grateful to the readers who will carry this work forward. I am excited about what we can transform together. May we journey with tenacity, integrity and patience.

CONTENTS

FOREWORD

At dawn, whenever I hear early morning birdsong, I am often returned to vivid memories of my childhood – my mother awakening at the *amrit velā*, the ambrosial hour before the sun begins to rise, and the sound of morning ablutions, *prāṇāyāma* and the recitation of prayers and mantra. My nose would fill with the scent of incense and then, when my mother finished her *sadhana*, the clashing of metal spoons and the smell of dhal bubbling away. All this before she set off to work in the iron foundry in the industrial heartlands of Britain. A cold, distant and hostile land to which she had migrated as part of the South Asian diaspora in the early 1960s. As a child, I would grumble at the old fashioned rituals and traditional practices – already assimilated into an all-consuming culture which defined my heritage as primitive, ignorant and backward. As I grew (wiser), I started to see the patterns of racism, hatred and division. I began to feel the impact of ancestral trauma. I began to understand that my rich culture and heritage had been stripped and stolen and that its value lay only in what it was worth to white people.

My parents were born as colonized children in the Punjab, India – they experienced the brutality of the Partition as the British Empire retreated in the face of a powerful Quit India movement under Mahatma Gandhi. Their elders had borne witness to the Jallianwala Bagh massacre at Amritsar in 1919 which became the pivotal point at which the "moral" argument for the British Empire in India failed completely. The spirit of the movement for independence was inspired and sustained in part by sacred texts, including the Bhagavadgītā and Gurbani, and spiritual faith and yogic practices.

I am descendant of the warrior heart of ancestors, elders and those of the land in India, a South Asian wisdom traditions holder and a yoga teacher. Yet it has taken me almost 30 years to find a yoga community in which collective freedom, justice and equity are the threads which weave and connect us together. 30 years ... of isolation, dissonance, silencing and exclusion. Underserved, under-represented, undervalued and under-resourced.

It has taken me all of this time to find a community in which the dominant cultural values of whiteness, and all that it signifies, are recognized, resisted and rejected. A community rooted in ethics, integrity and respect for South Asian wisdom practices, and the people of the cultural whole.

Dr Stacie Graham is an anchor within this community of yoga teachers, practitioners and dedicated change agents. She came into my world, like a comet, when Jonelle Lewis, our mutual friend, drew us, with Leila Sadgehee, into profound and deep conversations about the nature of systemic racism and the extent of cultural hoarding, harm and exclusion in yoga. As our philosophical values and lived realities in yoga became more visible, Stacie's critical understanding of the intersectionality of race and culture in yoga provided shape to our aspirations and commitments to create a force field of radical change.

In her skilful approach, Stacie crafts pathways to "doing the work" for trainee teachers and practitioners, to studio owners and proprietors and to influential brands. She provides tools to frame thinking into action. The practical and expert know-how that Stacie offers through her book is a labour of allyship to indigenous wisdom holders and an example of leadership to the yoga industry. This book honours the sacred gift of yoga while calling in responsibility and accountability to those with power, decision-making and influence.

The dreams that are possible to dream in yoga as exemplified by ethical businesses and studios included here in the book are, in Stacie's words, "so magnificent and beautiful and perfectly encapsulate what is possible in collectively created spaces".

For this "we must put in work – individually and collectively – in order to effect change ... It is genuine labour: labour of action, labour of love, grief labour ... this is the essence of yoga."

Thank you, Stacie, for lifting the practice and raising the bar for all those called and challenged to reflect, review and renew their commitments and actions to equity and justice in yoga.

Kallie Schut, decolonized yoga and dharmic traditions educator, founder of Rebel Yoga Tribe YouTube channel and the Radical Yogi book club

INTRODUCTION

HOW DID WE GET HERE:
THE INTERSECTIONS OF YOGA, CULTURAL
APPROPRIATION, RACIAL EQUITY AND
SOCIAL JUSTICE

My path to founding OYA: Body–Mind–Spirit Retreats was one of clarity, determination and disappointment. I must admit that it was not an entirely structured start nor planned in every detail. After completing my yoga teacher training in 2014, I travelled to Peru in 2015. I spent a part of that trip teaching *Yogāsana* in Cuzco. It was a horrible experience. I enjoyed spending time on the local markets, meeting and being embraced by Cuzqueños, participating in Indigenous ceremonies, and filling my belly with as many local dishes as possible. Simultaneously, I, the only Black woman on site, was continuously bullied from the moment I arrived by white women from Australia and the US who taught and resided alongside me. I often called a good friend of mine with tears in my eyes. As I am someone who does not readily cry in front of others, my friend knew that things must be bad. She is someone who is quick to offer unsolicited, often harsh advice. Yet in these moments she just listened.

After my stay in Cuzco ended, it took a while longer for me to recognize the learnings of these particular trials. However, by the end of 2015 I knew that I wanted to create a space where Black women and women of colour could congregate as they are. A place to share, to rejoice, to heal, to be. A place to reconnect with the Indigenous practices that historically have been forcefully removed from their lives. A place to attune to their bodies, a landscape upon which violence has for the majority – statistically speaking – been enacted. With scrappy tactics and wholly underfunded, OYA Retreats continue to build community with folks across Europe, Africa and North America.

The combination of the denial of freedom of movement due to a global public health crisis caused by the Covid-19 pandemic and the public and torturous murder of George Floyd proved to be too much in 2020, even for the ever reality-evasive yoga "community". Demands could no longer remain unheard and unaddressed. My network rallied, and I was contracted to work with a number of brands, yoga studio chains and teacher training schools to support their equity and inclusion efforts. The problem was that the majority were talking diversity, while I was only interested in equity. What is the difference?

Simply put, diversity is window dressing. Focusing on representation or the number of any given socially identified group does not mean much in the greater scheme of things. Especially if no other measures are taken to ensure that these underrepresented and underserved groups experience belonging while bringing their full selves to work, i.e., they will not thrive in these environments if nothing else changes. They will come and go; attrition rates for these groups will be high, but the numbers will look great for reporting to stakeholders.

In writing this book, I aim to provide some fundamental and easily implementable actions that can and should be taken by yoga teachers, studio owners, brands, as well as anyone else who actively participates in the so-called yoga and wellness industry. We each have a role to play.

BLACK WITH A CAPITAL B

Throughout this book, I capitalize the word Black when referring to people of African descent. Why? Because Blacks, like groups such as Asian, Latiné and other so-called ethnic minorities, make up a cultural group, and cultural groups are denoted with a proper noun.

If you don't know, now you know.

What Are We Here For?

My greatest motivator is to share what I have learned with a larger audience. I do not claim to have all the answers. I do, however, have tried-and-tested tools and practices to support folks in different phases of their unlearning journey.

Yogāsana has been co-opted and appropriated as fitness or exercise. The yoga industry in the United Kingdom alone is worth more than £900 million. That is US $1.208 billion. Even though much of the activity that is included when reckoning that total cannot be considered true to the wisdom tradition that is Yoga, much of it still carries the word or brand "yoga".[1] Given the size of just that one market, the potential impact of this industry to transform lives – as well as to cause harm – becomes clear. But do not let fear or thinking small lead you to believe that your actions cannot possibly change anything. Today, more than ever, individuals have the capacity to ignite movements and effectively demand change. There are countless examples of this occurring, both with the help of social media as well as through individual acts that catch on in different pockets of the world.

This book serves to nurture a community of change agents, who are committed to:

- acknowledging and honouring the origins of yoga;
- doing the work that is required of them to decolonize their thinking and unlearn harmful behaviour patterns;
- playing their part in advancing equity and creating justice in their yoga communities and beyond.

How to Use this Book

The book comprises four Parts:

- Part I. Tapas: Our Collective Path of Transformation
- Part II. Ahiṃsā: The Yogin's Path to Seeking Justice
- Part III. Asteya: The Leader's Path to Create Justice
- Part IV. Satya: Our Collective Paths to Freedom

Each Part is dedicated to particular groups that make up the yoga "industry". In the first Part, the foundation is laid for the entire book to create common ground through examining the explicit assumptions, expectations and historical contextualization of Yoga. Part II of the book is to support (aspiring) yoga teachers, specifically on their path to building and sustaining an increasingly inclusive teaching practice. In the third Part of the book, I turn to yoga businesses and their role in minimizing harm and abstaining from cultural appropriation, as well as advancing social justice and racial equity. Part IV, the final Part, ties the many threads together to illustrate how all these actors must come together to do better. In chapter 2, you can find a more detailed overview of the four Parts.

This book is written so that you can read it from cover to cover or you can flip to a chapter that interests you or pertains to your role in the industry. I would encourage you to treat the book as a resource to which you return again and again. It's not a "one and done", so there is no need to feel overwhelmed on the first read. It is not necessary to expect yourself to retain every action or step described. Instead, take out your highlighters, markers and sticky notes! The book asks of you to act, meaningfully and intentionally, which means you will likely need to return to chapters repeatedly for reminders of your next steps. With that structure in mind, some points are repeated in the relevant chapters to make it possible for you to start at any given chapter.

In each chapter you will find sections of displayed text: learnings, real-life examples and journaling prompts. The learnings are bits of information that I think are important to consider separately, without disrupting the flow of the text. Some of these address trending topics that regularly lead to heated discussions on social media or even in yoga classes. I keep them brief, and I encourage you to do your own homework. The real-life examples are offered as another access point into the subject matter. They are, of course, anecdotal, and I do not claim them to be the rule. Yet I hope they can make more tangible some of the discussion points that may be new or foreign to some readers. The journaling prompts are an important part of integrating the learning and making it more personal to your own experience. Keep your journal close by as you read the book and allow yourself plenty of unrushed and undisturbed time to write in stream of consciousness when prompted to do so.

What It Means to Do the Work

Over the last few years, there has been a lot of talk about "doing the work". That may annoy people for different reasons. For the love-and-light devotees, it may feel off-putting to refer to anything Yoga-related as work. Why? Because they preach that yoga is only about good vibes. The only work allowed is the kind that ends with an out. The anti-capitalist inclined may reject the invocation of work, because capitalist societies, in their view, have made everything about work and productivity.

And still, I stand by the fact that people need to do the work. I welcome synonymous phrases, such as going on the journey, being on the path, etc. However, it is important for all of us to recognize that there is work involved. We must put in work – individually and collectively – in order to effect change. The work I am referring to is not about force or simply going through the motions. It is genuine labour: labour of action, labour of love, grief labour, and others. This is the essence of Yoga. Some of you may be asking, "How sway?" Let us take it all the way back.

Back to the Beginning

In pre-colonial India, which includes the entire subcontinent, not just present-day India, the umbrella term *Hinduism* was not used to group different systems of thought together as it is today. Instead, you would simply refer to the various systems as Indian philosophy first, and then their specific identifiers; for example, *Vedānta*. The system of thought known as *Sāṅkhya-Yoga* is one of the oldest of these, but varying opinions abound concerning its origins. The order of coming into being and historical relation between the doctrines of *Sāṅkhya* and Yoga are unclear, their components being expounded by the authors Kapila and Patañjali respectively; however, their conception of the ideal life is fundamentally the same, while they differ in how to get there.

Sāṅkhya, a Sanskrit word meaning "reflection", describes the path to realizing the Ultimate through knowledge. Yoga, on the other hand, asserts that realizing the Ultimate is attained through steady and persistent meditation. It could be said that Sāṅkhya focuses on the theory, while Yoga sets forth the practical side of teaching. An understanding of the Sāṅkhya system is vital to a comprehensive understanding of Yoga. In the following discussion, however, we will home in on the foundations of Yoga.

The Yogic system comprises what are described as the eight limbs, petals, or accessories (*aṅgas*) of Yoga. They are:

1. *Yama*: abstinence, self-restraint
2. *Niyama*: observance, self-purification

3. *Āsana*: posture
4. *Prāṇāyāma*: controlling the vital force through regulation of the breath
5. *Pratyāhāra*: withdrawal of the senses
6. *Dhāraṇā*: concentration, steadying of the mind
7. *Dhyāna*: contemplation, meditation
8. *Samādhi*: total absorption, meditative trance

The eightfold path of Yoga can be regarded as falling into two phases. The first is about taming the will. The ethical code prescribed in the first two aṅgas supports the cultivation of virtuous behaviour. The yamas, which are directed toward the negative or restraining, include *ahiṃsā* (non-injury or non-harm), *satya* (truthfulness), *asteya* (abstention from stealing or misappropriation of others' property), *brahma-carya* (celibacy, sense control) and *aparigraha* (non-greed, disowning of possessions). The niyamas are positively directed and consist of śauca (purity), *saṃtosa* (contentment), *tapas* (right aspiration), *syādhyāya* (study of philosophic texts) and Īśvar-praṇidhāna (self-surrender, devotion to God).[2] The yamas and niyamas are the moral foundation upon which all Yogic training should rest if it is meant to be genuine and collectively beneficial. Practising breathing techniques and postures alone bears no spiritual fruit. The four Parts of the book are named after and based on the teachings from the ethical code of the yamas and niyamas. (More on that in chapter 2.)

The second phase of the path relates to the remaining six aṅgas and is fully devoted to the power and mastery of mental concentration and capacity. The first three – āsana, *prāṇāyāma* and *pratyāhāra* – cultivate controlling the physical body. The final three – *dhāraṇā*, *dhyāna* and *samādhi* – facilitate controlling the mind.

A dedicated and devoted practice necessitates sustained physical and mental exertion, i.e., work. Even at a first glance of the eight limbs, this is evident. And anyone who practises can attest to that fact as well. In addition, we live in a world of endless distractions and disruptions to our daily lives, of both internal and external origin. A world that, in recent history, has been built on the oppression of some groups to the benefit of others. To do our best in following the ethical code, practising frequently and consistently, and breaking the intergenerational bonds of oppression, we must work – and hard.

STOP GASLIGHTING WITH "YOGA MEANS UNION"

It is often stated that Yoga means union, but that is not the whole truth. The aim of meditation, or Yoga, according to the doctrine upon which the Yoga philosophy that travelled west is built, is not union, but separation. *Upaniṣadic Yoga* is a doctrine of union. Today's Yoga is one of disunion (*viyoga*).

The Upaniṣads are sacred scriptures that prescribe dhyāna – meditation. Several sections in the Upaniṣads describe modes of exercise, also known as *upāsanas*, which prepare the seeker for contemplation of the Ultimate. The aim of such contemplation is to develop the ability to fully grasp the unity of existence directly. To make such contemplation possible, an intellectual capacity and the detachment from selfish or self-centred interests are required. For this reason, Upaniṣadic teaching was meant to be kept secret and only conveyed to seekers or pupils who have gone through trials and tests to prove their conviction. The explicitly named concern was that offering such knowledge indiscriminately might lead to its distortion (welp!).

In the Upaniṣads, the individual self unites with or merges with the absolute Self through Yoga. However, in the system of thought known as Yoga, there is no such self acknowledged. Instead, the self comes into being by itself through disentanglement from *Prakṛti*, which can be understood as the origin of the Universe that is one and complex. Prakṛti is foundational to the Sāṅkhya.

If you don't know, now you know.

Why We Practise

In order for this book to really serve its readers, I believe that offering practice breaks is essential. Similar to the journaling prompts suggested throughout the book from chapter 1 onwards, the practice guidance offers you the opportunity to integrate what you have read. One step of integration is to recognize how things are landing in your body. In this context, "body" is a general term that includes the physical and mental aspects of ourselves, as well as our energy bodies.

Each practice is designed to meet at least some of the needs that may arise while doing the work that each chapter asks of you. At the same time, you are encouraged to practise outside of your reading journey. You may find that some of these practices resonate with you in particular situations or circumstances. Practice takes practice. So don't feel like you have to treat these as one and done. Come back to them again and again – without expectations – and notice how the experience shapes and re-shapes itself every time.

Before we move on to chapter 1, I would like to invite you to perform a body scan. Body scans are often associated with the practice of mindfulness. You may also encounter them at the end of an āsana class or in a *yoga nidra* practice, for example. It is not necessary to sit still or lie down to practise in this way. Any time you feel emotions such as joy, stress, grief or anxiety arising within you, a body scan is a useful way to observe where the sensations are strongest in your body. I chose to include a body scan here because it provides a foundation on which to build the other practices that are offered throughout. Furthermore, it can be supportive to use body scans as you read on as a form of non-judgemental exercise for checking in with yourself along the way.

Body scans in particular – and the practices found in this book more generally – alternate the awareness between narrow and wide frames of reference. This means that in the exercise on page XXII your attention will be brought to specific parts of the body before expanding to a wider view. Sometimes unexpected thoughts and emotions arise when we are asked to focus our attention in this way. If, at any time, your emotions feel too intense to bear or you experience strong physical reactions, such as breaking out into a sweat, then please discontinue the practice. Open your eyes. Take a few intentional and slower breaths. Connect to an anchor of your choosing, such as feeling your feet on the ground. Then take the time for something comforting like a cup of tea or a cuddle with a companion animal.

As described below, the practice guidance uses language referring to a non-disabled physical body. When I teach to groups, I adapt my language to the needs of the people in the space. I acknowledge that addressing a non-disabled physical body could potentially exclude approximately 15 per cent of the world's population. That is not my intention. The following instructions are invitational. I welcome adaptations to support your full participation in the practice.

Practice Break: Body Scan

Let us move into the practice. You can practise on your own or in a group.

Start by settling into a posture that feels comfortable to you. Sitting or lying down are comfortable options for this practice. If you choose to sit in a chair or on your sofa, place your feet firmly on the ground. Have the feet slightly apart so that your hips can relax. If your feet do not touch the ground, use a pillow or folded blanket to bring the floor up to meet you. If you choose to sit on the floor, sit on a cushion so that your knees are able to relax toward the floor. If you choose to lie down, you are welcome to lie on a yoga mat or even in your bed. Ensure that your head and shoulders are positioned so that the neck is not put under any strain. Place your hands slightly away from your body so that your chest can open with ease. Your palms can face upward for opening yourself up or downward for grounding yourself. For example, if you are experiencing physical tension in the body or are feeling resistant to the text, it may be better to have the palms face upward. If you are feeling nervous or anxious, you may choose to have the palms face downward.

Allow your body to settle. Notice if you need to make any final adjustments before coming into stillness. Be sure that you will be able to practise undisturbed for several minutes. You may need to close a door or turn your phone to silent in order to have the space to fully settle.

Soften the gaze or close your eyes, depending on your environment and how you are currently feeling. It is not necessary to have the eyes completely closed. In fact, if you are feeling tired or sleepy, you may want to keep your eyes slightly open.

Begin to bring your awareness to your feet. Notice any sensations in your feet: the arches and balls of the feet; the heels, the toes, the ankles. Sensations can be anything; for example, an itch, a sensation of cold or hot, etc. If it is easier you can start with one side of the body and then move to the other. Try not to judge if one side is easier to feel into than the other.

After you have explored your feet, bring your awareness to your lower legs – your calf muscles and shins. Observe any sensations in your lower legs.

In your own time, follow the sensations from the knees and then up to the thighs – fronts and backs. Observe any sensations in your knees and upper legs.

After you have explored your legs, bring your awareness to your hips, genitals and lower back. Take your time here to explore each of these areas. We tend to hold a lot of emotions in this part of the body. Take care not to judge or analyse anything you experience.

In your own time, allow your attention to move to the abdomen, chest and middle back. Here, where so many organs can be found, you may become aware of new sensations. Try to observe these with curiosity.

After some time here, move your awareness higher up to the neck, shoulders and throat. This is another part of the body where we accumulate and store emotions. Take care not to judge sensations – neither as good nor bad.

Take a brief trip downwards into the upper arms and elbows – fronts and backs. What are you able to notice here?

In another moment, allow your awareness to move into your forearms. What sensations are present?

Continue down into your wrists, fingers, hands – palms and backs. What sensations are arising? Do you recognize any differences between sides?

Allow your awareness to travel back up your arms and rest at your head. Tune in to each part: the back of the head; the jaw, mouth, tongue and teeth; your face; your ears; your hair. Take care not to judge sensations – neither as good nor bad.

As you prepare to allow your awareness to travel back down the body, you can do so with a supportive visualization, such as a warm light.

Begin at the crown of the head and allow your awareness to flow freely through the different parts of the body. In your own flow, move your attention from the crown of the head through the body until you reach the feet; and then move back up again to the crown. Do this at least three times.

When you're ready to continue, allow the light, or whatever you have chosen to visualize, to surround you. Spend some time, at least five minutes, fully present in this light.

At your own pace, begin to bring your awareness back into the space around you. You may want to first rotate your wrists and stretch your arms.

Take a few deeper, more intentional breaths.

In your own time, open your eyes or raise your gaze.

PART I

TAPAS: OUR COLLECTIVE PATH OF TRANSFORMATION

Across many faith and wisdom traditions originating on the Indian subcontinent, the word *tapas* can refer to any number of spiritual and self-discipline practices to tame the mind. It also refers to an inner fire or heated energy that supports reaching liberation or ultimate freedom. In this first Part of the book, I would like to invoke all the above. You may not view the next chapters as spiritual *per se*; yet I am making the case that the path of transformation is a shared one of patience and perseverance. It is a path that we do not travel alone, even if we desire to do so. And it requires a passion from deep within to continue, especially when things are hard.

CHAPTER I
SHARED LANGUAGE: AGREEMENTS AND ASSUMPTIONS

For many yoga teachers and practitioners based in Europe and North America, it may seem far-fetched to claim that Yoga is in any way related to current social justice movements. It is.

My understanding of social justice encompasses everything from criminal justice reform to transformative justice, economic justice, health equity and labour justice. Social justice means more to me than equal access to wealth, opportunities and privileges within a society. Social justice is the promise of every member of society being held up, being held accountable and simply being held. Social justice means that each member of society has the right to pursue self-fulfilment (individual) and Self-realization (relational) without being hindered in consequence of the multiple social identities they inhabit.

I could offer an analysis of much of the Vedas to make the case; however, that is perhaps another book for another time. Instead, I would like to point to just one key example, the *Bhagavadgītā*, often referred to as the *Gītā*, a 700-verse lyric that is a part of the great epic the *Mahābhārata*. The *Gītā* is, in the shortest description, a dialogue between a prince, Arjuna, and his guide and charioteer Krishna who is an avatar of Lord Vishnu.

Krishna captures the essence of the teachings of the Vedas through a discussion that touches on a range of spiritual topics as well as ethical, moral and philosophical questions. Throughout these teachings, Krishna makes clear that Arjuna, and people in general, must work with intention and persistence both for their individual liberation and for the stability of the world order. The *Gītā* is a text often taught on yoga teacher trainings, cited in readings and classes. Yet the spirit and meaning of the text has been replaced with "love and light" and other forms of toxic positivity. I define toxic positivity as the active resistance or ignoring of emotional, physical and mental pain that may be arising for someone in any given moment. There is an expectation to "rise above" that pain to embrace a positive outlook irrespective of the ability to embrace or experience positivity in the moment. Yoga does not ask of us to overlook and deny the realities of the nature of the world. Rather, it offers us the tools to face those realities with authenticity, courage, tenacity and compassion. As explained in the *Gītā*, Verse 50, "It is a mistake to think that pleasure is the aim of action. Pleasure is of a transitory nature. The real aim of action is knowledge. Through knowledge one attains detachment and ultimate freedom."[3] Our journey to ultimate freedom is individual and collective.

Agreements

In order for us to go on this journey together, it is important to ensure that we are working from a shared point of departure. As readers you are agreeing to the following:

1.   We acknowledge that we all participate – to our benefit and to our detriment – in systems of oppression. Globally, we are living in a society where certain groups of people are oppressed, and others have privilege based on that oppression. Oppressed, marginalized and minoritized people can have privilege. Members of a dominant culture can experience oppression. We allow space for a spectrum of experience. While the notions of dominance and oppression are not unique to any one culture or group of people, modern western civilization was built on the successful *industrialization* of oppression. As American author, professor, feminist and social activist bell hooks explains, the concurrent and convergent consequences of white supremacy, patriarchy, neoliberalism and imperialism mark most aspects of our lives. (In the Glossary at the end of this book, you can find definitions for these terms and more.) These terms may feel quite academic or even foreign for some; while others may feel especially well acquainted with them due to their real-life everyday consequences. Our affinities and opinions on everything from food, music, home, education, profession and beyond are touched by the world order and our place in it. It is impossible to disentangle them. But

it is also not necessary to disentangle them in order to change. In a world that has become increasingly globalized over the last four centuries, there are few parts of it that still remain in isolation.

2.   We recognize that we are interconnected and interdependent. We have personal responsibilities to the work of creating an equitable society. We each have our own unique purpose and part to play. What we do on the individual level feeds into the interpersonal. How we relate to the folks closest to us informs how we operate in society. We start with ourselves and then the work we do moves outward into our communities. We have the power through connection to shift culture. To change the different narratives of oppression dominant culture feeds us. We all have responsibilities to which we need to be held accountable. We can only do that through compassionate community.

3.   Even though the work is hard and uncomfortable, we are committed to doing it anyway. It is up to us to do the work to create the world we want to live in. At the same time, none of this is easy. We have to do it all the same. We have to choose connection over disconnection. We have to choose embodiment over disembodiment. We are willing to do things differently and sit with the discomfort that arises. We do not have to judge discomfort as "bad" or see it as an indicator that we are "wrong". We do not have to avoid the discomfort of not knowing. Instead, we can open ourselves to the learning opportunities that discomfort affords us.

4.   We understand that intention is not the same as impact. On this journey, we must accept that we will make mistakes. We must accept that, even when we are trying our best, we will communicate or act in ways that cause others harm. Instead of focusing on getting things "right", we focus on being present with our fellow humans. We do not have to fill the silence with justifications of why our intentions matter. Rather, we practise listening. Listening more than we speak. Listening with our whole bodies. Listening to understand, to support, to nurture, and to grow. So that when we apologize, it is genuine. We continue to learn. And we can always try again.

These agreements are bold. They help us to manage our expectations as we journey together. They remind us that we must be accepting of open ends. We may not find closure in the way that we normally do or want to.

This work is bigger than any one of us. And it will continue beyond our lifetimes.

OUR AGREEMENTS IN SHORT

1. We acknowledge that we all participate – to our benefit and to our detriment – in systems of oppression.
2. We recognize that we are interconnected and interdependent.
3. Even though the work is hard and uncomfortable, we are committed to doing it anyway.
4. We understand that intention is not the same as impact.

"WHITE SUPREMACY" AND OTHER TERMINOLOGY

As some terms have been introduced to the mainstream and, to some extent, misused or misappropriated across different media outlets, the value of the word or phrase can be diminished. I use the term "white supremacy" to denote an ideology that promotes a power-centred understanding of race, by which people racialized as white are considered inherently or innately superior to other races and should therefore dominate them.

Throughout this book, I use terminology that comes up in many settings. In the Glossary, on page 139, you can find the meanings I ascribe to those terms for the purposes of this book. I seek to use language that is clear rather than comfortable. I seek to use language that is invitational and allows space for different experiences.

JOURNALING PROMPTS

The journaling prompts in this book are an offering to support your work. Create a space so that you can journal with intention. That might mean returning to the journaling prompts at a time of day that better matches your creative rhythm, perhaps first thing in the morning or before you go to bed. Ensure that you have plenty of time – for example, five minutes per prompt – so that you do not rush your thought process. Use a journal that you can return to again and again. You will want it to reflect on what is a lifelong journey of unlearning.

» What reactions – physical, mental, and emotional – do words such as "discrimination", "bias" and "privilege" elicit in you?

» Where do you recognize your own privilege? Where have you experienced exclusion?

» When do you feel most uncomfortable with these themes? What would help you feel safer and more confident in such situations?

» What does an apology look like that resonates with you and supports a process of repair?

Naming and Addressing

Throughout the day we make many assumptions. This is an important brain function without which we would be totally overwhelmed before even getting out of the bed. Assumptions are useful; however, they can also create divisions and perpetuate bias. If you are a yoga teacher, you likely make assumptions about the people in your classes. For example, that the students want to be there because they like (or love) yoga. That seems like a nice assumption to make. But it does not leave much room for people who are present and have yet to find something gratifying about the practice.

To minimize the risk of assumptions becoming a source of disconnection, it is important to name things, including assumptions, as they become clear, so that they can be candidly addressed. This is easier said than done because, going back to the automated brain processes, we do not always recognize when our statements, our opinions, our forms of communication are based on specific assumptions. I want to name some of my assumptions (and hopes) for this book:

1. I assume that readers are reading from a place of genuine curiosity.
2. I assume that readers will disagree with parts and agree with others.
3. I assume that readers will understand that I cannot meet all needs in one book.
4. I assume that the content will be new for some readers and not enough for others.
5. I hope that readers will seek dialogue with me and other readers to continue the work.

IN REAL LIFE

To do the work we have to be able to relate it to our own lives. I hope that the "In Real Life" excerpts are useful in helping you integrate these topics into your own world. The following are two projects I want to highlight that demonstrate, with ease, how Yoga and social justice are interlinked. I also want to acknowledge that there are many more unsung heroes that you can get involved with in your local communities.

OmPowerment Project
This project's purpose is to create awareness for embodiment practices and trauma-informed Yoga in communities that often don't have access to such tools. As an example, one pillar of that work focuses on supporting refugees and other marginalized communities that have benefited from Yoga but whose access has been dependent on volunteer availability. Their mission is to promote community-

led leadership by offering refugee communities the capacity to lead themselves – teaching someone to fish, instead of feeding them for a day. By empowering these communities to lead themselves in the basic practices of self-regulation, these healing practices can continue regardless of volunteer skill sets and availability.

Prison Yoga Project

This project provides trauma-informed Yoga and mindfulness practices as a means of self-empowerment and self-rehabilitation.[4] On their website under the heading "Mission and Impact", they list several points that they address through their work, some of which are noted here:

- Develop the self-awareness, self-worth, empathy and compassion that leads to positive personal and pro-social choices.
- Foster a more peaceful and humane incarceration environment for incarcerated people and staff.
- Reduce the rate of recidivism among formerly incarcerated people.
- Assist prisons, governmental agencies, private entities and individuals in establishing trauma-informed Yoga and mindfulness programmes.

Loving-Kindness Meditation

In this chapter, I have only scratched the surface of what is an incredibly challenging subject. Words such as "bias", "discrimination", "oppression" and "privilege" often evoke strong reactions within us. However, we can no longer hide from these truths. Their real-life consequences serve as constant reminders why we must act, now. I know that for some readers this chapter is not enough. And again, for others this chapter may contain content that is new and, thus, feels overwhelming. There is room for all of those emotions and others. I encourage you not to allow fear and difference to keep you from reading on, or worse, from doing the work.

"The simple act of being completely present to another person is truly an act of love—no drama is required." These words from Sharon Salzberg's book *Loving-Kindness: The Revolutionary Art of Happiness* capture the reason

I offer this practice here. Even among yoga teachers and other wellness professionals, there will be cynics. It is important to make clear that I am not claiming that all problems of the world will be solved through meditation practice alone. Some institutions will have to go; others must be reinvented. The success of such grand transformations hinges on the willingness of the people to get the work done. To begin that work, we must build a consensus around, firstly, root causes of existing problems, and, secondly, the interventions that have the most potential to repair and rebuild. This work becomes possible when we are able to be truly present to (the needs, past hurts and future worries of) our fellow human beings and their communities.

Mettā is a Pali word that translates to "benevolence". Mettā refers to the type of love that is not steeped in desire. It is fully accepting of what is. It removes the origin of suffering – the feeling of separateness. In Buddhist meditation traditions, mettā practice is referred to as loving-kindness practice. Hatred and aversion, which are closely linked, are considered the opposite of the state of love, or mettā. The profoundness of a regular and consistent loving-kindness meditation practice, especially when doing this work, cannot be overstated.

Thinking about the enormity of the work ahead can feel crushing. When we focus our awareness on our neighbours, our peers, our friends, our colleagues, our family members and other loved ones, it feels perhaps even just a little more within reach.

Please be reminded that if you experience any form of distress, stop the practice immediately. Open your eyes and reground through your connection to your anchor.

Practice Break: Mettā Meditation

Let us move into the practice. You can practise on your own or in a group.

Start by coming into a comfortable seated position. If you are seated on the floor, take a cushion or blanket so that the hips are elevated, and the knees can relax toward the floor. If you are in a chair, place your feet firmly on the floor. If they do not touch the floor, put a cushion or folded blanket beneath them so that you can connect your feet to the Earth.

Allow yourself some time to settle. Notice if anything will disturb your practice. Take the time to change it and settle again.

Bring your awareness to your breath without trying to change or control anything about it. If focusing on the breath does not work for you, bring your awareness to your connection to the ground and the Earth.

Remain in a space of awareness for five minutes or so. It is normal that thoughts will arise. When you recognize that you are thinking, gently bring your awareness back to your breath or Earth connection.

Call into your awareness a neutral person. This is a person you do not know well, who does not evoke strong emotions. It is someone who you see regularly but do not know well. Greet them in a way that feels appropriate and consensual. Once you have greeted one another, express the following phrases to the person. This can be a verbal expression, or through some other visualized form; for example, through warm light.

- May you live free from fear.
- May you be free from suffering.
- May you experience joy.
- May you feel whole.

Once you have said or expressed the phrases slowly, say your farewells to the neutral person, so that they may depart with ease.

Reground through your seat and feel yourself connected to the Earth.

Call into your awareness a loved one, with whom you have a positive relationship in good standing. Greet them in a way that feels appropriate and consensual. Once you have greeted one another, express the following phrases to the person:

༁ May you live free from fear.

༁ May you be free from suffering.

༁ May you experience joy.

༁ May you feel whole.

Once you have said or expressed the phrases slowly, say your farewells to the loved one, so that they may depart with ease.

Reground through your seat and feel yourself connected to the Earth.

Call into your awareness yourself. Greet yourself in a way that feels supportive at this time. Once you see yourself before you, express the following phrases to yourself:

༁ May I live free from fear.

༁ May I be free from suffering.

༁ May I experience joy.

༁ May I feel whole.

Once you have expressed these phrases slowly, stay with the feelings that are arising within the body for a little while.

Reground through your seat and feel yourself connected to the Earth.

Call into awareness the community members of where you work and live. Greet them in a way that feels appropriate and consensual. Once you have greeted everyone, express the following phrases to the group:

༁ May you live free from fear.

༁ May you be free from suffering.

༁ May you experience joy.

༁ May you feel whole.

Once you have expressed the phrases slowly, say your farewells to the group, so that they may depart with ease.

Reground through your seat and feel yourself connected to the Earth.

Call into your awareness the communities by which you feel emotionally challenged. Try not to envision specific people. This is not meant to re-trigger experiences of violence or conjure people with whom you have had personal contact. Go bigger. Greet them in a way that feels appropriate and consensual. Once you have greeted them, express the following phrases to the group:

- May you live free from fear.
- May you be free from suffering.
- May you experience joy.
- May you feel whole.

Once you have expressed the phrases slowly, say your farewells to the group, so that they may depart with ease.

Reground through your seat and feel yourself connected to the Earth.

Call into your awareness all the Earth's human inhabitants. Greet them in a way that feels appropriate and consensual. Once you have greeted them, express the following phrases to the group:

- May you live free from fear.
- May you be free from suffering.
- May you experience joy.
- May you feel whole.

Once you have expressed the phrases slowly, say your farewells to the group, so that they may depart with ease.

Reground through your seat and feel yourself connected to the Earth.

Notice any bodily sensations. Remain here for at least another five minutes.

Allow the breath to deepen and become more intentional.

At your own pace, raise your gaze or open your eyes.

CHAPTER 2

HOW WE WILL WORK: CREATING TAPAS TO TRANSMUTE AND TRANSFORM

Sanskrit has played an essential role in conveying classical Indian literature. It is Sanskrit that delivered us the great epics of *Rāmāyana* and the *Mahābhārata*. Sanskrit is the language of the Vedas. The texts of Vedānta and Yoga were also handed down via Sanskrit. For this reason, we honour the language of Yoga in this book by using Sanskrit, written with the use of diacritics, as much as possible.

It is often argued in western yoga spaces that the use of Sanskrit is not inclusive. Some common arguments are that introducing a foreign language can feel alienating to students or expecting students to learn the words and phrases is a form of classism or elitism. However, I would counter by asking if the same would be true if I were including Greek and Latin terminology on a western philosophy course? Is it even feasible to imagine teaching philosophy, medicine or science without the use of Greek and Latin? The naming of SARS-CoV-2 variants reminds us that certain languages are considered universal, while others are relegated to ancient texts. What is the difference? If we want students and teachers to have an understanding of the cultural contexts of the practice they have come to learn, then we must include Sanskrit.

In the following chapter, I offer an overview of the four Parts of the book and how they are related to Yogic principles. There are journaling prompts to support your process of deepening the learnings of the principles as well as how they are relevant to current public discourse on Yoga and social justice. I recognize that many of these words are similar in other languages and dialects, such as Pali and Prakrit. However, I am focusing here on the most common meanings and translations from Sanskrit.

Tapas

Sanskrit: तपस्. The word *tapas* is based on the root *tap* (तप्), meaning "to heat", "to give out warmth", "to shine" and "to burn". Tapas means sustained practice and is the third niyama. As explained on page xx in the Introduction, niyamas are individual ethical observances or positive duties which complement the yamas.

The underlying notion of tapas is expressed in similar ways across different traditions. In somatics, it is said that to practise something 300 times creates muscle memory; to practise something 3,000 times leads to embodiment. Angela Duckworth describes in her book *Grit: The Power of Passion and Perseverance* how a combination of passion and persistence, i.e., 10,000 hours of deliberate practice – what she terms grit – leads to excellence or high achievement. In *Kriyā Yoga*, a system that consists of a combination of posture, breath, meditation, chanting and devotion practices in a fixed sequence, we also find that some sequences are recommended as a *sādhanā*, or daily spiritual practice, over 40, 90, 120 or even 1,000 days.

Tapas connects our outer practice to our inner transformation. Sustained practice is essential and works as a fire of change. However, the fire must not simply smoulder without developing the heat necessary to, for example, turn wood into charcoal, or turn our cognitive awareness into meaningful action for change.

The first Part of this book is linked with tapas. In these opening chapters, the foundation for the rest of the book is laid. One significant part of the root problem of injustice in the yoga industry is a general consumerist mindset. This mindset shows up in many ways. To take more than to give. To easily separate things into "I like this"; "I don't like that"; "I want this"; "I don't want that"; "this is good"; "that is bad". To mindlessly consume without questioning why. The term mindless here is used as the opposite of mindfulness. This type of "bread and circuses" serves as a distraction. We focus on the wrong things and fight with the wrong people, while oppressive structures keep us wanting for more of the same.

Maybe there is another way.

What does sustained practice look like? Stay true to the physical practice – āsana and/or kriyā for most – that introduced you to Yoga. There is nothing wrong with finding your access point through physical practice. As a next step, take the learnings off the mat. Notice how that euphoric feeling you sometimes experience on the mat arises when you move a little slower through your day, take the time to be present with others, cook food that is nourishing for your body, and get a good night's rest. Read books on Yoga that are not just about the physical practice and are written by non-white authors. Learn more about the origins and culture from which Yoga emerged. These are the types of acts that stoke the fire of change.

Ahiṃsā

Sanskrit: अहिंसा. The word ahiṃsā – sometimes spelled ahinsa – is derived from the Sanskrit root hiṃs, meaning to strike; hiṃsā is injury or harm, while a-hiṃsā, its opposite, is non-harming or nonviolence. Ahiṃsā is the first yama.

The yamas are principles put forth in Patañjali's sutras by which humans can strive for a soul-liberating freedom. The yamas, when heeded, are an integral part of Self-realization through self-restraint. The first yama, ahiṃsā, is likely the most cited in western yoga spaces. In many ways, this is a bitter irony as these spaces perpetuate a type of violence that many of us have yet to recognize as such – the violence of Eurocentric beauty standards.

To remove the origins and heritage of any wisdom tradition from the practice of it is a violent act. Against the backdrop of British colonialism that first tried to deny people access to their beloved culture and a present-day Britain in which people of South Asian descent are ridiculed and looked down upon for any clothing or customs deemed "traditional" while using that same clothing as a perfected festival costume, it is an act of violence to misappropriate and hyper-commodify one of the essential Indian philosophies.

If you search #yoga on any given social media platform, the likeliest top posts will include images of white women, predominantly dancers and gymnasts, in advanced postures, such as the splits or headstand. I have intentionally not used the Sanskrit words for those postures here, because the images are a show of acrobatics, not Yoga. The white women in the images are, mostly, very skinny, bendy and blonde. They are not representative of the general population. This, too, is an act of violence.

In the second Part of this book, I offer simple – not necessarily easy – ways that you, as practitioners and teachers, can minimize such harm with tangible examples to support understanding and unlearning. There is a saying that the path to hell is paved with good intentions. Let this be a reminder that even with the best of intentions, mistakes will be made. In our quest to minimize harm, we also have to be prepared to make genuine apologies. It is not possible to always get things "right". Release yourself from the hold of perfectionist desires and, instead, embrace the learning opportunities that arise in getting things "wrong". As Krishna warns those who mistake inertia for spirituality, "Neither let your motive be the fruit of action, nor let your attachment be to non-action."

BRITISH COLONIAL INFLUENCE ON (HAṬHA) YOGA

There have been a number of books on the origins of Yoga, including Susanna Barkataki's *Embrace Yoga's Roots: Courageous Ways to Deepen Your Yoga Practice*, so I will not dive deeply into that history here. What is important to note is, firstly, as mentioned in the Introduction, the understanding of Hinduism today is a grouping of differing schools of thought that British and European scholars forced upon the world during British colonial rule of the territory (1858–1947). Secondly, modern *Haṭha Yoga*, as exported to Europe and North America, was a response to British colonial rule.

Swami Vivekananda, who is credited with bringing Yoga to the west, aligned his teachings of Yoga – *Rāja* (the path of meditation), *Karma* (the path of action or good works), *Bhaktī* (the path of loving devotion) and *Jñāna* (the path of knowledge) – to the European Brahmin-centred interpretation of Hinduism. He arrived uninvited in Chicago to the World's Parliament of Religions in September 1893. He had two goals: to prove the worthiness of Hinduism to have a seat next to

Christianity, Judaism and Islam as a world religion and to bring attention to the crushing poverty his people were suffering under. Vivekananda had both half-accurate and, to an extent, bizarre notions of what Haṭha Yoga was. He viewed Haṭha Yoga as primarily focusing on fitness.

Within India, Swami Kuvalayananda worked tirelessly to prove through scientific experiments the physical and physiological benefits of Yoga. He founded the Kaivalyadhama Health and Yoga Research Centre and was editor of *Yoga-Mīmāṃsā*, a quarterly journal dedicated to publishing the findings of the Research Centre's experiments. Kuvalayananda sought to provide evidence to overcome the attitude of the majority of middle- and upper-class Indians – most of whom owned property, were well educated, and held a professional post under British colonial rule – who either dismissed Yoga as being irrelevant to their lives or looked down their noses at Yoga as a weird spiritual practice. Haṭha Yogins such as Kuvalayananda and Yogendra sought to promote the practice as a way to heal the body.

It should be mentioned that Vivekananda, Kuvalayananda and other Yogins of the late 19th and early 20th centuries identified as Hindu nationalists or, at least, shared their views. This must be seen in the context as a direct response to British colonial rule.

If you don't know, now you know.

Asteya

Sanskrit: अस्तेय. The word *asteya* is a compound derived from the Sanskrit language, where *a* refers to non- and *steya* refers to the practice of stealing or something that can be stolen. Thus, asteya means non-stealing and is the third yama.

There are overt forms of stealing, such as stealing physical objects. However, there are also subtler forms of stealing. Colonialist powers stole humans, land, minerals and more. And they deprived people of what is rightfully theirs – culture, dignity, language, honour and respect, for example.

How often have you said or heard someone say that they "invented" something in yoga? How often have you read something that misconstrues the influence of J.P. Müller's calisthenics system on contemporary Yogāsana practice? How many brands have you seen capitalize on words and phrases that have been introduced to the west through Yoga, even if Yogic principles are not a core part of their business or business model? These, too, are forms of stealing. It is not appreciation to claim ownership and domain over something that cannot be owned. It is not appreciation to seek to undermine a wisdom tradition that has continuously evolved over millennia. It is not appreciation to demean words or phrases that are sacred to wisdom and faith traditions.

In the third Part of this book, I provide guidance for yoga studios and teacher training schools, as well as brands. People have been calling out the issues that these organizations help to perpetuate for years. However, it took yet another senseless and cruel public murder of a Black man to get the attention of the mainstream. That attention may have been short-lived. Beyond some virtue signalling that took place during the protests of the summer of 2020, not much has changed in this industry. To create long-term and sustainable change requires us to take meaningful actions. In three chapters, we will turn to those actions in greater detail.

ON CALISTHENICS AND YOGA

There is a lot of misinformation on the influence of calisthenics on Yoga. This is a short-form description and position. J.P. Müller (1866–1938), a native of Denmark, created a modern-day calisthenics system. After being a sickly child, he went on to become celebrated in Denmark for amateur sports. In 1904, he published a home exercise book, *My System: 15 Minutes' Work a Day for Health's Sake!*, and it became an instant success. With this book, he hoped to address the common ailments of a growing middle class that, in his opinion, derived from stagnant and sedentary behaviour.

Yogendra (1897–1989), a native of Mumbai, had been a sickly and physically weak teenager. His health eventually improved, and he became a body sculptor. He was an avid reader and learned about the developments of physical culture in different parts of the world. One major influence of his youth was Müller's calisthenics system. When Yogendra went to study with his guru, Paramahamsa Madhavadasaji (the same guru as Swami Kuvalayananda's), he gave up body sculpting. After leaving his guru, Yogendra, similar to Müller, wanted to find ways to address the new and different needs of a growing Indian middle class that, from his perspective, suffered from ailments such as dyspepsia and obesity caused by increasing affluence.

Yogendra openly dismissed Müller's home workout system as "claptrap, charlatanry and pseudoscience". What he did appreciate about the system was its emphasis on short-form exercise. At the time, it was still common in Haṭha Yoga practice to return to its 84 āsanas. If Yoga should be made more accessible to middle-class Indians, then it would need to be practised differently. Yogendra created a routine called "The Perfect Course", which consisted of 13 āsanas, ending in śavāsana (corpse pose). The routine simplified previous Haṭha Yoga regimens and included *dynamic* variations. However, the dynamic system never caught on. It was criticized as impure or insufficiently challenging. Eventually, Yogendra even abandoned the dynamic variations.

Yogendra, recognized as the first Haṭha Yoga teacher by his biographer, left us with a legacy that majorly influences the way we practise today, including śavāsana at the end of class rather than *padmāsana* (lotus pose), shorter posture routines, and accessible class teaching. It is, however, Tirumalai Krishnamacharya (1888–1989) who fully instituted the shift from mostly seated to standing postures. It is well documented that the major influences of his standing and advanced posture practice came from street theatre performers in India.[5]

If you don't know, now you know.

Satya

Sanskrit: सत्य. *Sat* (सत्) is a common root word in Sanskrit. It means "that which exists", "that which is". *Satya* means "truthfulness". It is the second yama. Without the first yama, the second is not possible.

There are, for example, times where we may choose not to be *completely* honest with someone about what they are wearing or how they performed, because we do not want to unnecessarily hurt them or because we see that they are trying. Similarly, we do not beat the truth into people who are at the beginning of their learning journeys in any given subject. It does not work. We can watch how such tactics unfold every day on social media. To practise truthfulness with integrity, we must also practise nonviolence.

Because satya is firmly a part of the yamas, truthfulness is often positioned from a place of restraint. However, I would argue that it must also be positioned as an act to be truthful. Yama is a cultivation of the positive, not simply a suppression of the immoral.

In the final Part of the book, I address how to take this work forward. In delivering antiracism and equity and inclusion trainings, I have often received the feedback from participants that the experiential nature of the training made all the difference. For many of us, it is easy to read a book and think we've got it, we've understood it without ever relating it to our personal lives and experiences. Without the personal connection to our own work and actions, we are practising *dveṣa*, aversion. To continue to transform and evolve, we must look at the collective, as well as our own contributions to that collective, with discernment. Based on what we find, we must act.

JOURNALING PROMPTS

» What has sustained practice looked like in your life thus far? This does not have to be related to Yoga or wellness. Where have you been able to commit to a regular, or even daily, practice in the past? What kept you going? What prevented you from continuing?

> » To what extent do you practise nonviolence towards yourself? Where do you judge yourself harshly? To what extent do you practise nonviolence towards others? Where do you judge others harshly?
> » In what ways have you stolen – i.e., taken more than given – as a yoga teacher or otherwise?
> » How would you describe your commitment to acting truthfully?

There's Layers to It

This work can be understood across five dimensions: internal, interpersonal, institutional, structural and cultural.

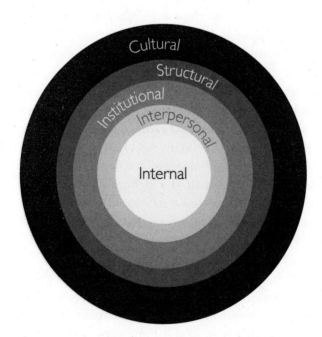

Above: An illustration of the relational dynamics between the individual and the collective.

Internal: the subtle and overt messages that reinforce individual and personal beliefs

Interpersonal: acts carried out from one person to another

Institutional: policies and practices that reinforce standards within workplaces and organizations

Structural: multiple institutions collectively upholding policies and practices

Cultural: shared knowledge, beliefs, customs, language, and other social behaviour among a group of people

Self and Collective Care – More than a Spa Retreat

"Self-care" has become a popular term. It is often used to advertise products and services that claim to make people feel good. Instead, they often make people feel worse, because they lead us to believe that self-care is something that can only be bought and sold. This narrative tells us self-care is a one-off, expensive, luxury experience that we can only afford ourselves every blue moon.

In these pages, I define self-care as intentional acts of care that can be integrated into daily life. Such acts have three ingredients: presence, intention and love. It is possible to practise self-care at any time of day and even when you do not believe yourself to be in the right state of mind. Self-care reminds us that we are more than our productivity and our output. Self-care nourishes the one true home that we have in this lifetime: our bodies.

There are many ways to practise self-care while reading this book and doing this work. For example, a daily gratitude practice can help internalize all that you value in your world, even when the world around you feels like it is in disarray. Positive affirmations can provide a light on the path of your aspirational self. Instead of "fake it till you make it", how about *say it – own it – be it*. I encourage readers to develop a self-care practice that allows you to tap into your own intuition and inner wisdom. A practice that helps you remove the barriers that prevent you from moving into relationship with others.

Without a well-integrated self-care practice, it is challenging to maintain a genuinely nurturing collective care practice. This is how we bypass the spiritual bypassing that often takes place in your favourite yoga studios.

If we are not taking care of ourselves, then we may find ourselves resentful when our collective care offerings are not reciprocated how we hope or expect them to be, or even at all. If we are not doing our own work, then it is not fully possible to be in relationship with others. Relationships become stagnant when parties are unequally committed to doing their own inner work.

At the same time, we must be careful that we are not hiding behind the "need" to do our own work. In Anglo-American societies, a phenomenon of hyper-individuality has developed. In the United States, this can be observed at every level from the individual to the institutional. As an example, grind culture wants you to have three successful side hustles all while getting your second online MBA and working a 9 to 5. Who and what does that lifestyle serve? When will you know that you've "made it" and can finally turn your attention to your communities?

Do not let fear get in the way of your leap from internal work to interpersonal. The internal work has no end destination. There is nowhere you must first get to before you can begin to do work in community. These journeys move on parallel and perpendicular paths. They cannot be neatly disentangled.

Why is "Transmute" Every Yogin's New Favourite Word?

I recognize that the word "transmute" has been enjoying a lot of attention of late in western yoga spaces. Maybe I should have chosen a different word; maybe not. I prioritize transmutation because it is not enough to simply "change". That change must come on several levels and in higher forms.

In history, we observe that change has often been led from the so-called bottom. Students and workers have been at the base of many of history's greatest movements. When it comes to equity and inclusion in organizational settings, I believe that there must also be momentum from the so-called top to make meaningful and sustainable change. It requires a suitable budget, so that employees doing this work are appropriately compensated, and it requires executive sponsorship to lend such work accountability and licence.

If enough organizations – of various sizes, business models, markets, and industries – make commitments to which they are held to account, both qualitatively and quantitatively, we create change that is not only institutional but structural. Similar to the internal and interpersonal dimensions, each organization has to commit to really doing the work of changing their own processes. Accordingly, these changes can be adapted and replicated in a way to fit the needs of specific markets and industries. Transmutation is achieved when a minimum number of organizations are on the same change trajectory, making bona fide structural change.

IN REAL LIFE

When Intentions Are Not Enough

The January/February 2019 issue of *Yoga Journal* was meant to be triumphant for people who do not fit the narrow Eurocentric beauty standards that westernized yoga has embraced. It was announced that Jessamyn Stanley, a Black, queer, self-identified fat woman, was to grace the cover. This was going to be a historical moment. And it was. But for the wrong reasons. The publication decided instead on a split cover: one with Stanley, and a second with Maty Ezraty, a skinny, white-presenting woman in an advanced posture.

The disappointment and outrage heard around the Internet was swift and fierce. Criticism was voiced by non-practitioners and practitioners alike. The message of the cover was clear: yoga is not actually for all. The publication reneged on a promise of change. It let fear of difference prevent it from offering Stanley her spotlight. It reminded Black women that the mainstream will never consider them enough.

If you are wondering what *Yoga Journal* learned from this incident, I would have to argue very little to nothing. In June of that same year, *Yoga Journal* offered Nicole Cardoza a cover and feature story. Cardoza is the executive director of Yoga Foster, a US-based non-profit that gives free and low-cost yoga training to educators. The story would feature the work that is being led by the organization. Shortly after the photoshoot with Cardoza, *Yoga Journal* ran a survey of three images of women against their typical magazine backdrop, asking audiences which one should be the next cover. The images did not include any words or further explanation. Cardoza was the only Black woman featured. All of this was done without Cardoza's permission or knowledge.

Cardoza reached out to *Yoga Journal* to ask their reasoning behind the survey. They replied saying that they needed to test potential sales. When she responded that she felt uncomfortable with their actions, she didn't receive any further comment from the publication. She posted about the issue on Instagram and received a great show of support. *Yoga Journal* did eventually make a reversal and give her the cover as previously agreed. As a form of repair, Cardoza had the magazine agree that all proceeds would go to her newly launched Reclamation Ventures, which gives grants to underestimated entrepreneurs who are working to make wellness more accessible.

The Power of Transformation

In this chapter, I have focused on transmuting and transforming the individual and the collective Self. The foundation has been set for the circularity of this work. It is individual, yet the individual is a part of the collective. It is neither possible nor desirable to disentangle the singular from the plural, the individual from the collective. However, in a world increasingly polarized, it can feel like an insurmountable, or even futile, act to try to cross divides and start a process of repair. An incredible amount of energy and will is necessary for us to maintain the endurance required to see work through that will not be completed within a single lifetime.

In the following practice, you are invited to bring your attention to the third primary chakra, or energy centre, known as *Maṇipūra* in the Vedic tradition. As for most Sanskrit words, the name Maṇipūra has a few different translations into English. Most commonly, it is translated as "city of jewels". The third chakra is located just above the navel, at the solar plexus. The colours associated with the third chakra are yellow, blue and red across the Vedic, Tantric and Nath traditions respectively.

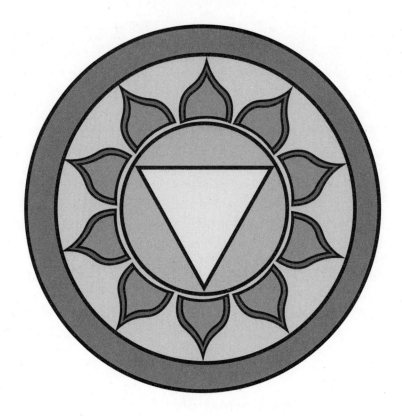

Above: Symbol commonly used for the third chakra, Maṇipūra.

Maṇipūra governs the digestive system; thus, it makes sense that it is associated with fire and the power of transformation. It is considered the centre of dynamism and will power. It is the source from which *prāṇa*, or flow of energy, is radiated throughout the entire body. In Kriyā and classical Haṭha Yoga, it is common to use different movement practices to arouse the energies in this part of the body. Further, there are similar concepts in a range of other wisdom traditions, such as *Kua* in qigong or *Hara* in some Japanese traditions.

In the following practice, you will activate the solar plexus region to tap into your fire, your power, your will. If for any reason you begin to feel unwell or stressed, end the practice. Open your eyes and anchor yourself through your connection with the ground.

Practice Break: Uḍḍīyāna Bandha

Let us move into the practice. If you want to experience the power of this practice, do it every day at dawn, or when you wake, on an empty stomach to realize its benefits fully.

To begin, take a standing position with your feet wider than your hips. Bend your knees slightly. If you cannot stand for long, then take a seated position in a chair, with your buttocks at the edge of the seat. Ensure that your feet are planted firmly on the ground.

Place your palms on the middle of your thighs, allowing the arms to bend slightly. Make sure the palms are on the thighs, and there is no weight on the knees.

Lower the chin towards the chest.

Inhale deeply. Open the chest by spreading the collar bones away from each other.

Exhale quickly through the mouth to empty the lungs.

Close your mouth. Hold the air out. Arch the back down as you would in cow pose. Don't let the chest become hollow.

Squeeze the abdomen towards the back. Maintain the abdominal grip without raising the chin.

Hold the grip for 15 seconds or as long as your endurance will allow. Don't overdo it! Build up over time.

Relax the abdominal muscles without raising the chin.

Inhale slowly. Take a few normal breaths.

Repeat the above cycle of inhalations and exhalations six times (see sequence below).

If you are standing, come into a comfortable seated position.

With the eyes closed or the gaze lowered, bring your awareness to the sensations coursing through the region just above the navel.

Observe, without judgement, the energy of the body. Take at least five minutes for this part of the practice.

At your own pace, raise your gaze or open your eyes.

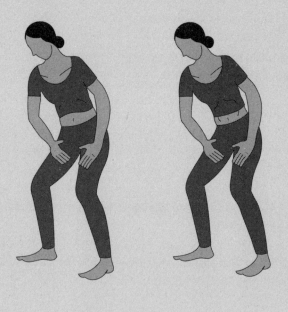

Let us now turn our attention to what we, as individuals and Yogins, can do to effect change.

PART II

AHIMSĀ: THE YOGIN'S PATH TO SEEKING JUSTICE

Ahiṃsā, the principle of nonviolence, is included in the first limb of Patañjali's eight limbs of Yoga. The first limb, yamas (self-restraints), together with the second limb, niyamas (positive duties/observances), make up the ethical code of Yoga philosophy. The first yama is ahiṃsā and refers to all living beings. As Yoga practitioners, we are to practise causing no injury to all life forms as a precursor to āsana, the third limb.

As humans, we must recognize that we will fall short of ahiṃsā, but that does not mean we allow ourselves to be content with only that which is within reach. As Yoga practitioners and teachers, there are many proactive and preventative measures we can take to ensure that we are doing all we can to minimize harm. And in the moments where we cause harm, we must be prepared to make amends. Part II points to actionable steps that teachers can take to uphold this principle in their teaching practice.

CHAPTER 3
THE 200-HOUR YOGA TEACHER TRAINING IS A RUSE

For most western practitioners, their introduction to Yoga is through the physical or posture practice, āsana. Āsana is described by Patañjali in the *Yoga Sutras* as the third limb of Yoga's eight limbs. Yoga Sutra 2.46 states that āsana means the posture that brings comfort and steadiness.

स्थरिसुखमासनम्

स्थरि-सुखम् आसनम्

Above: *Sthira sukham āsanaṁ*
Sthira = steady; sukham = comfortable; āsanaṁ = posture.

Each person will have a different access point into their own intuition and collective wisdom. There is no wrong way to access that which is universal and available to all of us. What is questionable, however, is the dominance of the physical and physiological in western yoga spaces. It reduces Yoga to an acrobatics or gymnastics practice through a teaching culture that is often predominantly mechanical. In contrast, C.G. Jung observed that, "In the East, where these ideas and practices have developed, and where for several thousand years an unbroken tradition has created the necessary spiritual foundations, Yoga is, as I can readily believe, the perfect and appropriate method of fusing body and mind together so that they form a unity which is scarcely to be questioned. This unity creates a psychological disposition which makes possible intuitions that transcend consciousness."[6]

For sure, many people attending classes are looking for a physical workout. In later chapters, we will look at the studio culture that promotes such expectations; however, in the next sections we turn our attention specifically to teaching culture.

I fully acknowledge that there are myriad reasons that may lead someone to choose to complete a teacher training. Not everyone who attends teacher trainings does so with the intention of becoming a teacher. Yet it is important to recognize that the teaching culture experienced in any given class has been cultivated by a combination of environments including the studios, the teacher training schools and the teachers with whom new teachers have learned. In my experience, most students are, to an extent, reproducing or mirroring their teachers' styles while still developing their own teaching style. Thus, the environment in which people train to become yoga teachers likely has significant impact on how they teach, at least at the outset.

Teacher Training – What's All the Fuss About?

According to its website, Yoga Alliance is the largest non-profit association representing the yoga community, with over 7,000 Registered Yoga Schools (RYS) and more than 100,000 Registered Yoga Teachers (RYT) as of April 2020.[7] While Yoga Alliance have announced that they are creating more pathways to certification, the standard path to becoming a registered yoga teacher is to complete a yoga teacher training at one of their registered yoga schools.

The standards for a 200-hour teacher training, the entry point into becoming a teacher, have recently been updated to put more emphasis on the ethics of yoga teaching as well as equity in yoga. However, the overwhelming majority of the 200-hour core curriculum, as prescribed by Yoga Alliance, is dedicated to the physiological–scientific–mechanical of teaching posture practice. One hundred per cent of the minimum 200 hours are classroom hours, i.e., in the presence of so-called lead trainers and faculty.

The British Wheel of Yoga (BWY) is the largest yoga membership organization in the United Kingdom, with over 7,200 subscribing members in 2015. It was awarded National Governing Body Status by Sports England in 1995. The BWY offers Ofqual-regulated, Level 4 teacher training qualifications. Ofqual stands for the Office of Qualifications and Examinations Regulations, a non-ministerial government department that regulates qualifications, exams and tests in England. Level 4 refers to the Ofqual system and is equivalent to the first year of a foundation degree, higher national certificate (HNC) or certificate of higher education (CertHE).

The entry-level teaching qualification with the BWY is a Certificate, which comprises five units (or modules) similarly positioning posture practice as well as anatomy and physiology as fundamental knowledge for teaching. Total qualification time is 290 hours, with 161 of those hours being in the presence of a tutor (lead trainer/teacher trainer).

We will get more into teaching schools in chapter 7, but there are a few questions you might want to begin asking yourself, your teachers and these institutions:

- How did 200 hours become the norm? Is this an arbitrary number or does it have meaning?
- How was the core curriculum crafted? Why is the physical practice emphasized above all other limbs?
- To what extent were wisdom seat holders of South Asian heritage centred in the process of creating the governing bodies? Why is that?
- How does a western credentialing system serve a South Asian wisdom tradition?

There are, of course, many other ways to train as a teacher that lie completely outside of the above-mentioned governing bodies. At the same time, it cannot be denied the outsized role that they play in training yoga teachers. The RYT and RYS trademarks indicate a certain level of standard, whether present or not in the teachers and schools respectively, and are globally the most widely accepted credentials in the yoga teaching industry. The same is true for BWY in the United Kingdom.

In the following sections, we will examine two examples of different teacher training pathways.

Bikram Yoga

Bikram Yoga is a system of hot yoga designed by the now disgraced Bikram Choudhury, an Indian man born in Kolkata who eventually immigrated to the United States in 1971. Classes consist of a fixed sequence of 26 āsanas and two types of prāṇāyāma practised in a room heated to 41° Celsius (105° Fahrenheit) with a humidity of 40 per cent. The sequence remains the same in every class, and every class should take exactly 90 minutes. At the height of his success, Choudhury stood at the centre of hot yoga practice.

In order to train in Bikram Yoga, a trainee only has to have been practising consistently and continuously for six months. A typical training takes place over nine weeks for a total of 200 hours and includes two posture classes per day, as well as lectures on yoga technique, osteopathy, anatomy and physiology. Further, trainees are taught a Bikram script to deliver to the class. This is key, because there are no hands-on adjustments, so the teacher must be able to vocalize the instructions rather than relying on hand placement. Certification is not guaranteed to everyone who attends. Trainees must be proficient in anatomy, the 26 āsanas and delivering the script.

The alleged verbal and emotional abuse as well as alleged sexual assault and harassment carried out by Choudhury on his students and faculty is well documented.[8] Further, he has faced accusations of stealing the āsana sequence from his own teacher.

Jivamukti Yoga®

Jivamukti Yoga® was "founded" by Sharon Gannon, a white American dancer and musician, and her partner David Life, a white American artist, in New York City in 1984.[9] The name is an adaptation of the Sanskrit term *jīvanmukta*, where the Sanskrit noun *jīva* means "life" and the past participle of the verb *much* or *muc* "to liberate". Together, it can be translated as freedom while still alive.

In contrast to much of westernized yoga, the Jivamukti method is comprised of five tenets: *Shastra* (scripture), Bhaktī (devotion), Ahiṃsā (nonviolence), *Nāda Yoga* (singing or chanting), and Dhyāna (meditation). In practice, however, the method is most known for its vigorous *Aṣtanga vinyasa* or flow-based āsana component, as well as the founders' ideologies of veganism and environmentalism.

On their website, it is claimed that the Jivamukti Yoga® Teacher Training is the most comprehensive training course available. There's one pathway to becoming a Certified Jivamukti Yoga Teacher, which requires over 400 hours of study and includes an introductory course, a foundational course (75 hours), as well as the actual certification course (300 hours). Some of the prerequisites for registering on the foundational course, where their spiritual warrior sequence is taught, include having taken a minimum of ten Spiritual Warrior classes over the previous six months and reading a bunch of publications by the founders. The comprehensive certification also prioritizes āsana, with other limbs and practices primarily serving as supplementary to āsana.

The founders, as is custom in South Asian wisdom traditions, often express gratitude to the South Asian teachers and masters with whom they learned. They studied across the *Sivananda* and Astanga traditions as well as with one of the most well-known Indian gurus, Swami Brahmananda Saraswati, also known as Guru Dev, among others. It is, thus, striking that so much of their teaching and publications are in their own names. How can one claim to own a wisdom tradition by trademarking a combination of Sanskrit words and publishing the truths that were conveyed orally by Indian sages? How can one claim to be different from the mainstream when actions illustrate the same possessive and colonized behaviour as the rest of the field?

David Life, Sharon Gannon and other senior teachers faced allegations of abuse of power.[10]

What these training programmes share is an excessive reliance on certification. Yoga teacher training certification processes, as the phrasing suggests, are created to indicate a level of standard with the hope that students will experience little difference in the quality of learning āsana. Instead, students will choose their teachers based on chemistry, resonance and connection. Modern science is obsessed with the notion of standards, paradoxically without questioning the arbitrary nature of said standards.

To honour the fact that āsana is not merely a gymnastics or dance class would mean that attending classes for a few months would not suffice as a prerequisite to register for a teacher training. It would also mean that a significant amount of time is spent on studying sacred texts, such as the *Bhagavadgītā*. However, in a colonized world the wisdom derived from ancestral transference is looked down upon as inferior knowledge or even quackery. Modern medicine is quite belatedly coming to recognize the scientific rigour of, for example, *prānāyāma* as known to Indian sages, documented in Taoist writings dating back to 400 BC, and embodied in practices of First Nation and Native American peoples. To build teaching standards that detach posture practice from its greater purpose of calming the mind and turning inward is serving neither teachers nor their students. It does, however, serve making money because it allows for faster growth. (More on that in chapter 7.)

IN REAL LIFE

My Journey to Teacher Training – Attending a Yoga Alliance International School[11]

I played sports at a competitive level from the age of eight. During that time coaches focused primarily on an athlete's performance, i.e., output and achievement. After suffering a recurring injury, I continued to play sports and weight train for my mental and physical wellbeing but not to compete. Eventually, I began to have other symptoms that, after a lot of tests and doctor visits, were found to be due to the hardness of my muscles, specifically in my neck and shoulders. It was the first time I had ever heard that hard muscles could be harmful. A close friend of mine, who is a qualified physical therapist, recommended I start practising yoga.

After about five years of regular yet infrequent practice, I visited India for the first time. I had always wanted to visit South Asia, as a part of my studies were seated at the South Asia Institute of the university where I received my first degree, but I never found the opportunity. Again, a good friend of mine suggested that I take a much-needed break from writing my doctoral dissertation and spend at least three months in India. He was originally from Mumbai and helped me plan the first part of my trip.

It was at the foothills of the Himalayas in Rishikesh where I met new friends and had the privilege of experiencing *satsang*, or a gathering together for truth, in the presence of many profound lineage and wisdom seat holders. Even at the International Yoga Festival, which is hosted at Parmarth Niketan – an ashram in Rishikesh – each year and includes many white western Yoga teachers, I recognized what had been missing in my previous classes back at home: a connection to something beyond physical practice.

After returning from India, I knew that I would like to deepen my practice, and I knew that I needed to go back to India to do so. With the help of my new friends-for-life, I was able to identify a few teacher trainings that were led by Indians and targeted predominantly local populations. The Yoga teacher training I decided on took place in Sikkim and included in its curriculum Buddhist philosophy and meditation. The curriculum was taught by three teachers from West Bengal and a Tulku Rinpoche originally from Tibet. There were five trainees from western or European countries, including me. The rest of the trainees were from different parts of India. And it was very clear, even in intense and awkward moments of white fragility, that the teachers prioritized their students from India. I was thrilled and felt at home.

JOURNALING PROMPTS

» Why are the people completing trainings not representative of all parts of society?

» What systems enable white people to offer trainings in South and Southeast Asia with little to no local representation among their trainees or teaching faculty?

» What made you decide to train as a yoga teacher?

» What characteristics were most important to you in a school when you decided to complete a teacher training? To what extent did your choice fulfil those expectations? What would you do differently today?

» How do you define your sense of purpose in teaching yoga?

POWER DYNAMICS OF THE TEACHER

Any curriculum to train teachers is remiss if it does not address positionality and power dynamics. This is an essential subject especially in consideration of the wave of allegations of abuse of power that has rocked yoga and other wellness communities across North America and Europe. This entire book is asking you to reflect on your (social) location and the role it plays in your relating to a wisdom tradition with roots in South Asia. Here follows an overview to get you started.

It starts with you: often yoga teachers invest a lot of energy in building their capabilities to teach to different abilities, bodies and proficiencies that show up in a general class. Similarly, teachers must build a capability of self-awareness of their location in society. The realities of racism, sexism, classism and more shape the composition of and interaction within yoga classes just as they do in wider society. That means that every teacher must work to understand how their multiple social identities overlap and interplay with those of their students.

Reflect on Your Social Location

Below is a table to help you locate yourself, both in the ways that society has ascribed to you as well as your own self-claimed identities. There is no wrong or right way to complete the table. It is completely up to you and may change as you continue on your own path of learning and un-learning.

PARENTS	
Race / Ethnic Background	
Formal Education Level	
Income (growing up)	
Language Spoken at Home	
Citizenship Status	
Relationship to Mental & Physical Health	

SELF	
Age	
Dis-/Ability	
Gender / Gender Expression	
Complexion	
Sexual Orientation	
Formal Education Level	
Native Language	
Religion	
Passport / Citizenship	
Occupation / Profession	

Holding Power

Power is a nuanced and challenging subject for most people. The simplified version in the context of this chapter is that in your role as a teacher you are in a powerful position. The power of the yoga teaching role is amplified because Yoga has the potential to be a heart-opening practice.

You do not know what histories and presents sit before you in the shape of your students. No matter how long you have been teaching them, you do not know what they are carrying in their bodies and minds. To respect these dynamics requires, above all else, humility from the teacher. As a teacher, you are not meant to know everything. You are not meant to be without imperfections. You, too, are human.

When students make you aware of discomfort or harm caused through your facilitation, then it is time to pause. Not defend but pause. To listen. To ask how to support the student, how to repair, or how to make amends.

JOURNALING PROMPTS

» What does it take for you to acknowledge a mistake or forgive a mistake?

» What does accountability look like to you?

» What do you need in managing conflict to move forward with a better understanding?

Earth Grounding Practice

In this chapter, I have begun to highlight just how multi-layered the discussion on advancing equity and inclusion in the yoga industry is. Teaching culture is an important pillar in changing the industry, as teachers are the face of Yoga in most practitioners' experience. If the industry relies on a colonized certification process to train the next teachers, then it becomes clear how existing systems are easily replicated without that needing to be the intention. As a teacher, you may also feel encouraged to find that there is an opportunity for you to actively and definitively contribute to changing a multibillion-dollar industry in ways that create meaningful impact almost immediately.

The following practice uses breath and minimal visualization to bring the Earth's stabilizing and grounding energy into the body. The practice will support your downloading and integrating what may have come up for you in this chapter, for example through the journaling prompts or even the social location table. We have to be intentional in creating space for the physical body to absorb new information, to recalibrate so that new information moves from a cognitive to an embodied understanding. The practice can be taken in stages. When you are short on time, you can choose one part of the practice that serves you in that moment.

Practice Break: Earthing

Let us move into the practice. If you have access to an outdoor space, you are encouraged to use it. However, this practice can also be done indoors. If it is not possible to stand, the practice can be undertaken in a chair. Your eyes can be open, lowered or closed throughout.

To begin, take a standing position with your feet comfortably apart so that your lower back feels supported. If you are outdoors, be sure to take your shoes off. If you are indoors and wearing socks, take those off.

As you stand, allow the shoulders to descend toward the ground while your arms relax by your sides. You can turn the palms to face forward, or they can remain facing the body without touching the body.

Lift your toes off the ground, spread them as wide as you can, stretch them away from the feet, and then place the toes back on the ground. The intention of these actions is more important than great movement.

Bring your awareness to the feet. Ensure that the feet are grounding through five points — the upper outer edge (at the base of the small toe), lower outer edge of the heel, lower inner edge of the heel, upper inner edge (at the base of the big toe), and the centre of the arch. Try to spread your weight evenly across all four corners and arches of the feet.

Root through your feet into the ground and allow your spine to extend into its natural curve.

Allow the breath to deepen as you breathe into your length, feeling into the roots of the Earth just like a tree does. Extend simultaneously through the feet and the crown of your head. Feel into the deep sense of security that is possible with stable and deep roots.

After some time, breathe into your width as a way to tap into the expansive nature of the body – both physical and energetic. Be reminded through that expansion of the vastness yet interconnectedness of life.

Feel the stable and steady energy of the Earth support your expansion into your length and your width. Root through the Earth as you soften to the rhythm of nature.

Allow any arising thoughts, sensations or feelings to flow through you and exit through your feet, giving over their attachments and challenges to the Earth.

Remain here as long as you would like. When you are ready, end the practice with an expression of gratitude – even more powerful if vocalized – for the Earth and nature.

Let us now explore easily implementable changes to your teaching practice.

CHAPTER 4

MINIMIZING HARM: THE MOST MARGINALIZED MATTER EVEN IF THEY ARE NOT IN THE ROOM

One of the most common reasons that people offer to explain away their inaction is some version of "but we just don't have that many [insert social identity category] in our area". In most cases this is not the complete picture. But the focus of this chapter is not to argue numbers or statistics; it is instead to make the case for something often overlooked.

In understanding the needs of the most marginalized people in society and, in turn, responding to them with appropriate and compassionate solutions, we create products, spaces, jobs and much more that are inclusive to everyone in society. Let us repeat that again: if the needs of the most overlooked members of society are met, then everyone's needs are met.

This is the fundamental difference between equality and equity. Equality is defined as equal access to tools and opportunities. The underlying assumption that would guarantee equality leads to fairness is that all humans are equal (accurate), and all those equal humans have the exact same needs (inaccurate). Take, for example, an entrance to a building. The building has only one entrance. Anyone wanting to enter or exit the building must use the same door. At first glance that looks fair. There are no VIP or secret entrances that give people special access. However, on closer inspection we notice that there are a few steps at the entrance. This – at first – fair "one entrance for all" policy will actually fail many people who, for one reason or another, cannot get past the barrier of steps.

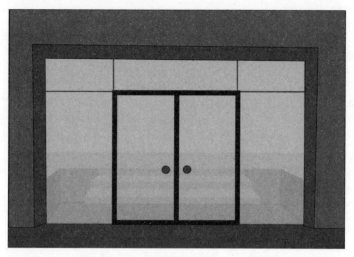

Above: An example of a building that has one entrance for everyone entering and exiting the building to use.

In reading this example, it is likely easy for you to identify why there is a need for change, which could come in several forms: for example, to add a second, barrier-free entrance; to remove the barriers at the current entrance; or even to add a ramp or some other provision to make it possible to get past the barrier. These examples are solid; however, they only address one aspect of overlooked needs. We must ask more questions to uncover further needs. One of those questions would be: how many people use the entrance at any given time of day? The answer may help us determine if there are times where people cannot access the entrance with ease, if the traffic needs to be directed, if the limitation to one entrance is a potential fire hazard, and so forth.

This example serves as a reminder that we must remain curious and ask questions. We cannot simply rely on what is visible or known to us. It also illustrates that we so often don't know what we don't know.

Gatekeeper or Door Opener

One hurdle to this type of reflection can be an unwillingness to receive. That unwillingness comes in many forms. It may appear as defensiveness: "I can't be held responsible for everyone else's problems." It can show up as blame:

"It's not my fault; it's so and so's fault." It might look like self-righteousness: "I have taught for X years, and I have never had anyone complain." Or it could even surface as a comparison: "I'm [insert social identity category] and confronted with discrimination every day, but it hasn't stopped me."

All of these are common, but that does not make them any less insidious. To what end are these statements used, if not to simply defend, deflect and invalidate other people's experiences? As yoga teachers, you have the tools to attune to your body's responses to feedback. You have the tools to meaningfully reflect and appropriately adapt your previous way of teaching to respond to the current needs of your students and our times. In the words of Toni Morrison, "The function of freedom is to free someone else."[12] In your role as yoga teachers specifically, this is your assignment. Have you understood it?

JOURNALING PROMPTS

Either referring to your answers from the previous chapter or starting anew:

> What made you choose to do that first teacher training? What did you hope to learn?

> Think about your original reason/that final push to train and compare that to your sense of purpose as a teacher now.

> Can you remember what drew you to your first teachers? What was it exactly?

> Have you ever received evaluations on how students experience your classes? If so, what stood out? What did you change?

Sri Yogendra, who is credited with teaching the first Haṭha Yoga class on a beach in Mumbai on Christmas Day in 1918, understood the needs of the people whom he aimed to reach. A new middle class had established itself in urban areas. They were benefiting from increasing monetary wealth yet poorer physical health. He changed the environment in which Yoga had been previously taught to meet their needs without sacrificing the integrity of an ancient wisdom tradition.

- ✻ What shifting needs have you identified since the beginning of the Covid-19 pandemic?
- ✻ What did you learn during the protests of the summer of 2020?
- ✻ How have you integrated these shifts into your teaching practice? If you have not yet integrated them, what is keeping you from change?

Yogendra recognized that having to travel to hard-to-reach hermitages and ashrams would keep the people from the practice who needed it most. Similarly, you must ask yourself what is keeping people from your classes and what lies within your power to change that.

Question Your Assumptions

Let us explore two scenarios that are taken from the real-life experiences of people I know.

IN REAL LIFE

The Unnecessary Use of Gendered Language in Classes
A teacher, who identifies as a cis-woman, was teaching a general yoga class. In it, she spent an extensive amount of time speaking from her personal experience of parenting. (All good so far.) She went on to make the statement that the most powerful act a woman makes is birthing her child. To paraphrase, childbirth turns a mere woman into a powerful woman. (How did we get here?)

At first glance you may ask yourself wherein the problem lies. Women face sexism every day. In some rich countries like the United States, women, and more generally parents, are not even afforded a decent amount of paid time off after childbirth. That is all true. It is also true that pregnancy and childbirth are experiences that are not

---

limited by gender. People of all genders can get pregnant and birth children. People of all genders can menstruate. Just as people of all genders may, for a variety of reasons, not menstruate or experience childbirth.

In this particular example, a cis-woman was present in the class who suffered from infertility. After several rounds of fertility treatments, she was forced to give up her dream of conceiving a biological child. She was heartbroken. The teacher's statement in a general yoga class, a place she least expected the subject to come up, left her devastated. So devastated that she did not return.

Many people have only recently begun to explore gender and gender expression, and how these are influenced by a Eurocentric patriarchal view of gender roles. If we, as teachers, have trans, intersex and non-binary students front of mind in crafting an active teacher vocabulary around gender, then we are, simultaneously, ensuring that people who for medical, personal, social and other reasons fall outside of so-called gender "norms" are not excluded either.

Hands-on Adjustments and Consensual Touch

Depending on what form of yoga you teach, you may or may not have strong opinions about hands-on adjustments.

In this next example, a student was participating in a general yoga class taught at a studio that she regularly attends. She was still recovering from an injury and was happy to be back practising in a studio setting. The teacher leading the class is a popular teacher known for his hands-on adjustments. At the beginning of class, he neither asked students about injuries nor did he seek consent to touch them. (We are not off to a very good start here.)

As the class progressed, the teacher eventually made an unsolicited adjustment on the student. Before she had the chance to decline or protest, he had made the adjustment in the exact physical region of her injury. She left the class re-injured. Moreover, she blamed herself for the pain, because she felt that as a teacher herself she should have been able to advocate for herself more clearly and proactively.

She eventually found the courage to make management at the studio aware of what had happened. The studio reacted defensively and blamed her for not responding in the moment. After some back and forth, the teacher did conditionally apologize for what happened while claiming that the student, too, needed to own her role in the injury.

Had the student had a visible injury or disability, do you think this scenario would have happened in the same way? There is a myriad of reasons why someone may not want to be touched in class. These may have to do with conditions, such a post-traumatic stress disorder, or be as simple as a student having eaten garlic at lunch. No matter the reason, students deserve to have a choice. No matter how well you know the student, they deserve to have a choice every time they step onto the mat in your class.

These are two examples that I hope have inspired and challenged you on the things that you take for granted and the assumptions you make in a class. Take some time to journal about other assumptions you make about your students and how this affects the way you teach. A good example: you likely assume that your students enjoy and want to be in a class if they have paid money for it. But that may not be the case!

A Safer Space for Teachers and Students to Fail

परणिामतापसंस्कारदुःखैर्गुणवृत्तविरोधाच्च दुःखमेव सर्वं वविेकनिः॥२.१५॥

परणिाम ताप संस्कार दुःखैः गुण वृत्ति वरिोधात् च दुःखम् एव सर्वम् वविेकनिः ॥

Above: *Pariṇāma tāpa saṁskāra duḥkhair guṇa vṛtti virodhāc ca duḥkham eva sarvaṁ vivekinaḥ*

50

Yoga Sutra 2.15 serves as a reminder that life is painful (keeping in mind that pain must not equate to suffering). It is painful because the material world is separated from the spiritual world; i.e., the material world cannot offer everlasting happiness. Thus, its experiences feel painful. If we can learn to detach from the cravings or desires imprinted upon us through the three *guṇas* (see Glossary), we experience less pain. As yoga teachers, there is a propensity to attach to our being liked or loved by students. When receiving feedback that may feel less affirming or more critical, a teacher attached to sentiments of approval and validation is likely to lash out or feel disgruntled. If your teaching practice can be separated from selfish motives, then your teaching vision can find a purpose that does not rely on uncritical devotion to be happy.

Harriet Minter, at the time editor of the *Guardian*'s Women in Leadership, delivered a talk once at a TEDx Women event in Whitehall where she described her experience in a yoga class as a "safe place to fail". While it is not possible to *fail* in a yoga (āsana) class, because showing up, stepping on the mat and moving as your body will allow *is* the practice, the sentiment of safety, especially psychological safety, is an important one. Psychological safety, simply defined, refers to an environment in which people feel they can bring their full selves into the space. A space in which all ideas are welcome; all questions are encouraged; all mistakes are addressed with care and compassion. A space in which each person has complete freedom to be, as long as that freedom does not infringe or threaten the freedoms of anyone else. In reading that definition as a yoga teacher, it becomes evident how conducive psychological safety is to supporting students in advancing their practice. Ensuring that your teaching practice does not merely tolerate or accommodate the most marginalized, rather it embraces and honours them – irrespective of their presence in the space – is fundamental to psychological safety.

Mettā Practice

I will be suggesting a mettā or loving-kindness practice to support the integration of the work you have begun in this chapter. Mettā is a way to overcome the illusion of separateness. That illusion lies at the centre of oppression, of othering, of feelings of isolation and alienation. Through mettā practice, we are reminded that we are all connected. As set out in chapter 1, the work is individual and interpersonal. The individual work is essential, but it is not enough. It is essential to recognize what subtle and overt messages – helpful and harmful – you have internalized and how they show up in your teaching practice. Mettā practice can support cultivating a shift in those messages that manifests in more compassionate interactions with your students and, more generally, fellow human beings. Tuning in to that connectivity can support your letting go of the desire to sit in a teacher's seat in which you are all-knowing and infallible. It can support your moving toward co-creating spaces with your students in which it is ok to make mistakes, be held to account, and develop a shared path of amends.

Loving-kindness helps us accept our humanness. It also reflects back to us the areas in which we are not kind to ourselves. This can be a powerful exercise if we are able to allow ourselves to sit with those reflections. We may begin to bring up our inner obstacles to expressing and accepting what is.

As you move through each stage of the practice, begin to observe where resistance to the practice shows up in your body. Observe without judgement of what is good or bad, right or wrong. Simply notice the body's response at each stage.

End the practice immediately if you become especially stressed or notice any major changes in your heart rate or breathing patterns. Open your eyes and anchor through your connection to the ground.

In the following, a short practice to cultivate kindness and connectedness is outlined.

Practice Break: Mettā

Let's move into the practice. You can practise on your own or in a group.

Start by coming into a seated position that feels comfortable to you. If you are seated on the floor, take a cushion or blanket so that the hips are above the knees, and the pelvic floor, hips and knees can relax.

Bring your attention to your breath without trying to control its depth or rhythm. If your breath is not available to you at this time, bring your attention to where your body connects to your seat.

Remain in this space of awareness for the next five minutes or so. As thoughts arise, bring your attention back to your breath or your body.

Call into your awareness a neutral person. This is a person you do not know well, who does not evoke strong emotions either way. Greet them in a way that feels appropriate and consensual. Once you have greeted one another, express the following phrases to the person. This can be a verbal expression or some other form – visualized through rays of light, for example.

․ May you experience joy.
․ May you be healthy.
․ May you live a life free from fear.
․ May you feel your connectedness to all of humanity.

Once you have said or expressed the phrases slowly, say your farewells to the neutral person, so that they may depart with ease.

Re-ground through your seat and feel yourself connected to the Earth.

Call into your awareness a dear friend with whom you have a positive relationship in good standing. Greet them in a way that feels appropriate and consensual. Once you have greeted one another, express the following phrases to the person:

․ May you experience joy.
․ May you be healthy.
․ May you live a life free from fear.
․ May you feel your connectedness to all of humanity.

Once you have expressed the phrases slowly, say your farewells to your dear friend, so that they may depart with ease.

Re-ground through your seat and feel yourself connected to the Earth.

Call into your awareness yourself. Greet yourself in a way that feels supportive at this time. Once you see yourself before you, express the following phrases to yourself:

🕊 May I experience joy.
🕊 May I be healthy.
🕊 May I live a life free from fear.
🕊 May I feel my connectedness to all of humanity.

Once you have expressed the phrases slowly, stay with the feelings that are arising within the body for a little while.

Re-ground through your seat and feel yourself connected to the Earth.

Call into awareness the people who regularly enter spaces you create or classes you teach. Greet them in a way that feels appropriate and consensual. Once you have greeted everyone, express the following phrases to the group:

🕊 May you experience joy.
🕊 May you be healthy.
🕊 May you live a life free from fear.
🕊 May you feel your connectedness to all of humanity.

Once you have expressed the phrases slowly, ask the group to create a circle.

Call into the circle the people who are missing from the spaces you create and the classes that you teach. Ask them to create a second circle in the middle of the first circle. Greet them in a way that feels appropriate and consensual. Once you have greeted everyone, express – together with the people in the outer circle – the following phrases to the inner circle:

🕊 May you experience joy.
🕊 May you be healthy.

❧ May you live a life free from fear.
❧ May you feel your connectedness to all of humanity.

Once you have expressed the phrases slowly, ask the group to expand the circles so that everyone is connected through one circle. Look around the circle and connect with the people present for a little while.

Say your farewells in a way that allows everyone in the circle to depart with ease.

Re-ground through your seat and feel yourself connected to the Earth. Notice any bodily sensations. Remain here for another five minutes.

Allow the breath to deepen and become more intentional.

At your own pace, raise your gaze or open your eyes.

CHAPTER5

LEARNING HOW TO LEARN: STAYING RESOURCED AND CONTINUING YOUR EDUCATION

Part II of this book aims its attention at teaching culture and the role that teachers play in creating inclusive environments in which everyone can thrive. I recognize that these chapters are too short to cover every possible scenario you may encounter as a teacher. For this reason, in this chapter we turn our attention to staying resourced as you continue on your path of transformation.

Present-day education systems vary according to country and culture. However, the majority share the model that the teacher is meant to teach, and the student is meant to learn. Teachers have all the knowledge, and students' existing knowledge is of little relevance. These roles are clearly delineated. In order to succeed within such a system, the student must simply play back or reproduce what the teacher has said. The student does not have to believe it or even understand it. The student's skill lies in correctly identifying how to win the game, i.e., pass tests.

Most yoga teacher trainings are similar. Trainees do not necessarily have to believe or understand the curriculum. They simply need to memorize the musculoskeletal system, replicate the delivery script of the trainers, and contort their bodies into the postures being taught.

Maybe there is another way.

For teachings to endure, they must resonate within the people receiving them. For teachings to resonate, they must be fully developed yet offer enough space and freedom for the universality and simultaneous uniqueness of humankind. The *Yoga Sutras* and the *Bhagavadgītā* are two examples of sacred teaching texts that are both universal while speaking to the specificity of the human experience. These texts cannot be memorized and then quoted indiscriminately. They are too precise, too distinct. Instead, they require time of the reader. Time to process. Time to reread. Time to integrate into the understanding of everyday circumstances. These texts also bring us back to an essential function of education: learning how to learn.

A Decolonized Approach to Critical Thinking

Who do you follow on social media channels? It is well documented that we build our echo chambers by following personalities and friends who agree with us. This can express itself as white female yoga practitioners, for example, following folks who look like them. The intention behind the question is to provide an impulse for people to begin to follow folks who don't look like them and don't necessarily share their perspective. There is, however, so much (junk) to sort through across social media, so what is so bad about just sticking with what is familiar?

One common concern I hear from students is that they feel overwhelmed with choice, and there is a particular anxiety that arises in making the wrong choices when trying to get things right. Marginalized and minoritized people reiterate time and again that we are not a monolith. If you follow five Yoginis of South Asian heritage, you will find great diversity of thought. This will be similar for any group of minoritized people, just as it is for members of dominant culture. The human desire is to find that easy fix, the one book or podcast or social media profile that offers all the answers. And with those answers, you will never have to worry again about making a mistake, because so-and-so said so. This is the type of learning that the education system set us up for. But we have to move through the discomfort of uncertainty and accept that for most things in life, and especially in deconstructing systems of oppression, there is no black and white. There is no easy fix.

Maybe there is another way.

I would like to offer a model of critical thinking. Critical thinking, as a discipline, may conjure associations of "logic", "rationality" and "scientific rigour". Those terms may feel intimidating to some, invigorating to some and oppressive to others. The following model is offered more as a type of framework to move through as appropriate. Autonomy remains with the user. The only consistent is that the user will remain in that fuzzy grey area.

RIED

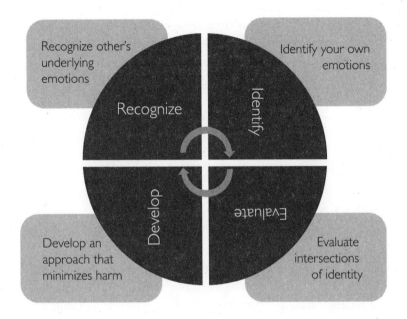

Above: The RIED four-stage critical thinking model for a reflective approach to managing conflict and building consensus for equitable and inclusive solutions.

Pronounced *rēd*, this four-stage model is cyclical rather than linear. It may be that you move forward on a continuum or have to go back a step after finding new answers. The cycle may even need to be repeated several times, even for the same event or circumstance, due to the number of parties and competing interests involved.

Recognize

Recognize others' underlying motivations. Without understanding these, or at least trying to, you may come to the wrong conclusions. What may prove challenging in this step is that what people say is not always the whole truth. That is not necessarily malicious or manipulative. Depending on their own practice, they may or may not have access to what is driving their actions in any given moment.

For example, if you were in conversation with a studio owner/manager and discussing the lack of *visible* diversity in one of your regular classes, you might ask yourself such questions afterwards:

♣   Was the owner listening?
♣   What was the owner's breathing pattern?
♣   What did the owner's body language communicate about their state of presence?
♣   How long have they been running this studio?
♣   How has the discourse shifted since they opened it?

These types of questions provide context. Context is important; however, our perceptions and interpretations of context are greatly influenced by our personal positionality and location in wider society.

Identify

Identify your own assumptions. In any given moment, we are all working under particular assumptions. It is a necessary function of survival. The brain has to make thousands of decisions every day. Without assumptions, the brain would be overwhelmed by the time we finish brushing our teeth after waking. At the same time, we need to slow down, in critical moments, to identify the assumptions upon which we are leaning.

Sticking with the example above, you might ask yourself some of the following questions:

♣   How do I typically relate to the owner?
♣   How well do I know the owner?
♣   How comfortable am I with this subject?
♣   Did I feel I was able to convey my message clearly and easily?
♣   What surprised me in this conversation? What does that say about my expectations going into the meeting?

If you find yourself in a reactive state, it is better to pause and ground yourself before asking yourself these questions. If time and distance are not sufficient for you to settle, you may want to talk it out with someone who you trust to simply listen, rather than offer feedback or advice.

Evaluate

Evaluate the intersections of social identities. This step is integral to the model as well as to finding new ways to work and engage that do not replicate the systems of oppression which cast a shadow over every aspect of our lives. Power is built into the social constructs of our identities because *dominant* culture, both subtly and overtly, has established what is deviant behaviour and what is acceptable (the norm).

At this stage, you may find that it becomes necessary to re-visit the previous stages with the insights gained here. Relying on the original example, your perception or analysis of the conversation will change depending on:

- your race/ethnic background versus the owner's race/ethnic background
- your gender and gender expression versus the owner's gender and gender expression
- the language in which the conversation was held and how that relates to your and the owner's first language
- your role as an employee/freelancer/other stakeholder of the studio
- your race/ethnic background in relation to the race/ethnic background of the visibly missing students (or gender, disability, etc.)

And the intersections don't stop there. Keep in mind that intersections are not inherently one-way hierarchical streets. This stage notably calls for the practice of sitting with discomfort and abiding in the grey.

Develop

Develop an approach that minimizes harm. Through society's norms and the role of rewards in our education systems, we have been trained to seek neat boxes of perfection, where everything can be tidily filed into categories of our choosing. This is harmful. The extent of that harm goes beyond what is experienced daily in yoga and wellness spaces.

To minimize harm, we must first acknowledge that it is possible to cause it, even in a yoga or wellness space. Reciting empty phrases of "love and light" and "yoga means union" causes harm. Conflict avoidance causes harm. Acting out of fear causes harm. Actions steeped in the desire to look *not racist* cause harm. Taking up space rather than making space for those who have historically been denied it causes harm. Justifying detrimental impact with good intentions causes harm.

Instead, we have to let go of the desire to file things and people away in finite categories. We must remain humble so that we are listening more than we speak. We must practise patience in the middle of paradox.

In an article for the *Washington Post*, American civil rights advocate and leading scholar of critical race theory Professor Kimberlé Williams Crenshaw explains that, "The better we understand how identities and power work together from one context to another, the less likely our movements for change are to fracture."[13] With the above framework, I am not offering a cookie-cutter recipe to learning and effecting change. The REID critical thinking model demands of its users an openness to self-enquiry, compassion and experimenting. You may not complete the exercise with a definitive answer; however, you will have learned something. Take that learning forward. Change does not come all at once. It comes with patience, perseverance and practice.

Mindfulness of Thought

In this chapter, I have offered a perspective on how education systems have primed us for a narrow model of learning. For the learning and unlearning that is required of us to decolonize our yoga (teaching) practice, the REID critical thinking model introduces a dialogue between the cognitive, the emotional, the conditioned and the experienced. Unlike many critical thinking models, there are no perfected decision trees or arrow models that lead to one clear answer. That may feel unsatisfying.

We spend one-third to one-half of our waking life not living in the present. We think somewhere between 6,000 and 65,000 thoughts a day, and this model is asking us to think more! We cannot stop thoughts. The mind is meant to think in the way that the heart is meant to beat. We can, however, develop a wiser way of working with our thoughts, so that they may slow. So that we are not consumed by our thoughts or ruminating for an extensive amount of time on negative experiences. In the same way that, in wiser relationship with the heart, we are able to slow the heart rate in times of fear or anxiety.

The following practice can be understood as a meditation on mental processes. In developing mindfulness of thought, it becomes possible to work better with REID, including in the moment as a conversation or encounter unfolds.

Practice Break: the 3Rs

Let us move into the practice. You can practise on your own or in a group.

Start by coming into a seated posture that feels comfortable to you. If you choose to sit in a chair or on your sofa, bring your feet firmly to the ground. Have the feet slightly apart so that the hips can relax. If your feet do not touch the ground, use a pillow or folded blanket to bring the floor to you. If you choose to sit on the floor, use a cushion so that the knees are able to relax toward the floor. Your palms, placed comfortably on your thighs, can face upward for opening or face downward for grounding.

Allow your body to settle. Notice if you need any final adjustments before coming into stillness.

Soften the gaze or close your eyes, depending on your environment and how you are currently feeling. It is not necessary to have the eyes completely closed. If you are feeling tired or sleepy, you may want to keep your eyes slightly open.

Bring your awareness to your breath as an anchor for attention. Do not try to control or alter the breath. Simply allow yourself to rest in the awareness of your breath. If your breath is not available to you in this moment, bring your awareness to your connection to the ground.

After some time, open your awareness to the sensations of the body.

After a while, further open your awareness to the sounds around you. If this becomes too much or too distracting, reduce your field of awareness to the sensations of the body.

Observe your patterns of thought – without judgement.

Notice that thoughts will continue to come and to go. Observe the nature of your thoughts without judgement and without attachment.

Release each thought and bring your awareness back to your sensory landscape.

Recognize the thought. *Release* the thought. *Return* to your anchor or the sensory landscape of the body.

Thoughts are just thoughts. A thought of what you plan to cook for dinner is not the meal itself. Can you see that?

Observe the impermanence of thoughts. How does it feel to come back from being lost in thought? How does it feel to think rather than to be lost in thought?

Notice the nature of your thoughts and how these connect to emotions and the sensory landscape of the body. If, at any time, thoughts begin to overwhelm you, bring your awareness to your anchor.

At your own pace, begin to bring your awareness back into the space. You may want to first rotate your wrists and stretch your arms.

Take a few deeper, more intentional breaths.

In your own time, open your eyes or raise your gaze.

Let us now turn our attention to what the collective – studios, teacher training schools and brands – can do to effect change.

PART III

ASTEYA: THE LEADER'S PATH TO CREATE JUSTICE

Asteya, non-stealing or not misappropriating what belongs to others, is the third yama. There is generally not a lot of time spent on this yama on yoga teacher trainings. There is a tendency to focus on the first yama, ahiṃsā; however, it could be argued that this is the most important yama to integrate into training, practice and the business of yoga teaching.

One's understanding of stealing will change as one continues on this path of unlearning. As children, we learn the most obvious of such moral or ethical principles. Do not steal toys from friends. Do not steal items from stores. For the majority, that is easy enough to uphold. In the realm of social media, though, lines become blurred. People, intentionally or unintentionally, steal quotes or phrasing, choreography, viral posts and even ideas. Who can say where an idea came from once it has circulated across three different social media sites? These examples may still seem obvious to some readers.

Misappropriation is more challenging. As we do this work, the subtlety of stealing shifts, making it easier to identify what *qualifies* as misappropriation, who normally benefits and who normally contributes without credit or compensation. The role of organizations is becoming increasingly more important in preventing and/or minimizing this type of harm. Socially conscious end consumers demand it of them. Over the next three chapters, studios, teacher training schools and brands are offered tangible steps to do better.

CHAPTER 6

STUDIOS: KNOW THE BUSINESS IMPERATIVE

How many headlines have you read referring to the "business case" for diversity, equity and inclusion (DEI) efforts? How many times have you heard a CEO or other business leader announce the steps they are taking to "diversify" their boards, senior leadership teams and general staff? How many times have you yourself, as a studio owner or manager, acted with haste to hire someone who identifies as Black, or a person of colour, to avoid being called out for doing too little? While these statements may appear to have the best of intentions, let us unpack some of the barriers ingrained in them that limit our path to true equity.

Let us begin with the word diversity. The *Merriam-Webster Dictionary* defines diversity as "the condition of having or being *composed* of differing elements, especially the inclusion of people of different races, cultures, etc. in a group or organization". As the definition makes clear, diversity should be used to define the composition of a group; i.e., a group can be diverse. However, the term is often misused to state that a person is diverse. A person cannot be diverse. Adding a person, who is considered different or an outlier, to a group of people, who are considered the same, does not create diversity. This is not mere semantics; this informs how we think about and approach diversity efforts. As studio owners, you are not being asked to add one person to your teaching, front of house or business team who does not look like the rest of the team. You are being called upon to completely reshape the composition of your teams and organizational culture.

The issue with the business case is less straightforward. Let us take it in two parts: harnessing diversity and the business imperative as an argument.

Harnessing Diversity

While there have been a number of empirical studies published over the past two decades that claim to provide evidence on the benefits of diversity, this research is largely unsubstantiated and inconclusive. Firstly, these studies define diversity in different ways, making it difficult to design a meta-analysis. (A meta-analysis is a statistical analysis that combines the results of multiple scientific studies.) The meta-analyses that have been published in peer-reviewed academic journals found no significant relationships between *mere* diversity and performance.[14] Some studies focus specifically on women, without taking into account other social identities such as race, sexual orientation, and parental status. Some studies include "women and people of colour" without observance of an intersectional approach, which means the experiences of people who identify as both are captured singularly either in the women category or in the people of colour category, and sometimes not at all. And again, other studies mix even more social identities under the hub of diversity and include people who identify as lesbian, gay, bisexual, trans, and/or queer (LGBTQ+), people with disabilities, and so forth. More issues ensue; for example, that not everyone who identifies as LGBTQ+ or as a person with disability is out at work. Moreover, without an intersectional approach, a white gay man's experience cannot be compared with that of a disabled woman of colour of any sexual orientation. In the best case, these studies exhibited correlations rather than causalities. But even in those cases, many of the studies carried out by consulting firms do not stand up to scientific rigour.

Further, it cannot be expected that simply adding people to a team or organization *automatically* leads to greater financial performance. There is enough research to demonstrate that an inclusive culture – a culture in which people of differing identities and thoughts are empowered to thrive – is fundamental to improved outcomes. If teams are tokenizing their "diversity hires", then there will be a high turnover of such hires, as they will have a higher likelihood of being bullied and/or suffering from burnout, or be among the first to be dismissed in an economic downturn. To leverage and reap the full benefits of a diverse workforce requires creating a team culture that celebrates and encourages different ways of working, that cultivates listening, that redefines power, thus shifting power dynamics, that reimagines and makes transparent performance recognition and reward, and that proactively addresses and makes space to negotiate conflict.

The Business Imperative

For decades, business literature thoughtlessly repeated phrases like the "legal, moral, social and economic" cases for diversity, equity (equality) and inclusion. And, admittedly, I have reiterated them, with intention, in my writings and on my website while (im-)patiently waiting for journalists and leaders alike to catch up. The legal case is the business case. The moral case is the business case. The social and economic cases are the business case. You cannot separate an organization's legal duties from its business. Previously, giants in industries such as tobacco, oil and gas happily separated their moral obligations from their business offerings. Today, many would say the same about tech companies. As studio owners, you likely rebuff any comparison to companies in the aforementioned industries. What connects all business owners is the fact that, in this new age, end consumers demand more. There is no need to separate these arguments because they all lead to the business imperative (and can be denoted in monetary terms for those of you for whom that is helpful).

The more insidious issue arises in linking the value of DEI efforts with financial performance. Is the argument then that such efforts are only valuable in the case that they improve financial outcomes? Does that give businesses the right to discontinue pursuing these goals if their financial forecasts are not met within a specific timeframe? Is it possible that linking the value of DEI programmes to financial performance leads to more bias, rather than less? And where does that leave those stakeholders – employees, (activist) investors, end consumers and others – who genuinely prioritize the social impact over the economic benefit? Can socially conscious stakeholders support these programmes in good faith if their value is being tied to financial performance alone?

Doing the Work

Yoga studios have a critical role to play in transforming the yoga industry to reflect the values of the wisdom tradition from which it was born. Marginalized members of the wider yoga "community" have been calling for change for years. It was not until the collective outcry after George Floyd's murder that some studio owners began to listen. Others proved remarkably resistant to the social justice protests of the summer of 2020. Black squares were hurriedly posted on 2 June 2020 for #Blackout Tuesday, but what happened after that? Very little. With a common excuse of financial viability, most studio owners went back to life as usual once the collective sense of urgency had receded and new headlines were formed. It is important to acknowledge that people frequenting studios expect more from them. This is the nature of a business that is built on creating and enabling wellbeing for its patrons.

JOURNALING PROMPTS

» What is your understanding of diversity? How diverse is your business (taking into consideration staff and patrons)?

» What barriers – material and nonmaterial – have you identified that may keep people from visiting your business?

» What marketing channels do you use to reach people? To what extent are your marketing materials representative of everyday life?

» How is your space decorated? To what extent are your decorations conducive to creating an inclusive environment?

» What extras do you offer at what prices? Are your vendors and their supply chain representative of wider society?

Yoga studios, gyms, and other wellness spaces of all sizes need to take meaningful actions to create long-term change. For example:

Resources: Set up resources specifically for DEI work and create a budget. Pro tip: attach the budget to your revenue so that the budget for DEI work grows with the growth of your business. Hire experts to come in and support this process, rather than expecting your existing staff members to do it without dedicated paid time or other compensation.

Metrics: Let both qualitative and quantitative data tell the story. You do not know the extent of your shortcomings because you have perhaps never measured it appropriately. You were likely content with feedback from a narrow or small audience.

Commitment: This work begins with senior management. If senior leaders in your business do not understand or prioritize the work, then there's little hope for change.

Training: Senior management need training in antiracism as well as other to-be-specified themes aligning to your organization's DEI programmes.

Processes: Create processes across the needs defined and measurable goals set. This will be the foundation for shifting a culture that previously did not prioritize equity and inclusion.

More training: Offer trainings for staff leading these new processes so that they embody and champion this new set of values. Measure engagement and receive feedback on every training. Keep in mind that trainings are not one and done. You will need to create learning experiences that evolve alongside the development of the business.

Reflect: Measure change/progress against the baseline from the beginning of this process (see *Metrics*, above).

Repeat: DEI is not a race to win. It's not a destination to arrive at. Repeat these steps for many, many cycles – especially the trainings, which may come in many forms. Unlearning is harder than learning, and there is a bunch of unlearning to do.

This may read simple, but it is not at all easy. You will encounter resistance from within yourself and across your business every step of the way. This type of process is new to most people in senior positions in wellness spaces, and your first response may be defensiveness. That may look like grumbles of "this isn't new to me", "we've tried women-only classes, and no one came so we stopped again", or "you don't know/ understand our business". Once you have had an opportunity to sit with and release that resistance, you will find a great tool to use with your team in the next section.

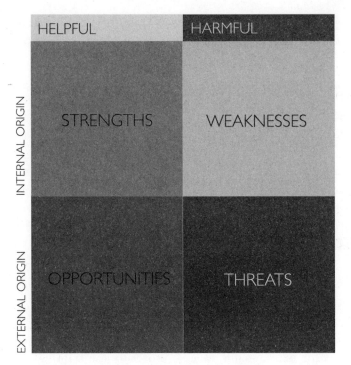

DEI SWOT

	HELPFUL	HARMFUL
INTERNAL ORIGIN	STRENGTHS	WEAKNESSES
EXTERNAL ORIGIN	OPPORTUNITIES	THREATS

Above: The four parts of a SWOT table.

A SWOT analysis is a strategic planning tool that has been used by organizations for decades. This type of analysis helps business leaders identify their strengths, weaknesses (or, as I like to call them, development needs), opportunities and threats. A SWOT analysis is best utilized in the early stages of decision-making processes. The DEI SWOT analysis functions by supporting people and organizations in creating their DEI strategy, and it serves as the foundation for the DEI matrix.

If you own or manage a studio, an important exercise in supporting the steps from *Metrics* through to *Processes* described above would be to collate a DEI SWOT. It would be useful for you to identify how different groups – for example, teachers, front-of-house staff and head office –

would complete the analysis. Rest assured there will be differences among those groups. Frame the analyses around the following questions:

> » **S**: What strengths in advancing equity and inclusion does the studio or space [insert appropriate name or space here] already demonstrate?
> » **W**: Where do current needs lie to better/further advance equity and inclusion at the studio?
> » **O**: What opportunities await the studio through measurably delivering on an equity and inclusion strategy?
> » **T**: Where do threats lie in doing that work? *And/or.* Where do threats lie if the studio does not do enough to address equity and inclusion?[15]

After completing the SWOT analysis, the next step would be to create a DEI matrix to distil what the next steps may look like with respect to improving on strengths, leveraging opportunities and minimizing the potential harm of current weaknesses.

IN REAL LIFE

Interview with Haji Healing Salon

Below is a written interview that was provided by the founder and owner of Haji Healing Salon, Aya-Nikole Cook, in November 2021. Haji Healing Salon is based in Chicago, Illinois in the United States and is a vibrant space for transformation activated by healers, mystics, teachers and therapists, with the shared intention of inspiring and supporting people on a healing path.

What was the catalyst for opening Haji Healing Salon?
I honestly feel my whole life has been the catalyst. I think it's relevant to say I have always been a very sensitive person. As a child I was hyper-aware of the suffering of others, and I was so impacted by it that my parents attempted to shelter me from certain environments and experiences they knew would challenge me. There was suffering within my family, though, and they couldn't shelter me from the sickness and addiction that plagued many family members. I remember feeling so powerless in the face of the pain I witnessed. It made me more religious. I was born into a Buddhist family, so I took refuge in the practice and spent lots of time praying for others and studying to better understand the way out of suffering. When I was 16, I began exploring other spiritual practices and moving toward vegetarianism in the hope of preventing illness. By then, I had become what most would call a "hypochondriac". The hyper-empathy I didn't understand at the time had morphed into full-blown health anxiety.

When I was 18, I met my first guru or spiritual teacher (outside of Buddhism). Jalil was a Black man, a yogi, massage therapist and herbalist. I took up an intense apprenticeship with him for three years and felt empowered by all I was learning. As I continued on my path, I encountered many spiritual teachers who contributed to me. My most significant teacher, however, was the illness I was diagnosed with when I was 27 years old.

When I learned my uterus was filled with fibroid tumours, I understood I was being invited into a deeper self-study: I was vegan and spiritual, living a healthy lifestyle. How and why did this happen to me? Because of the tumours I began practising yoga in earnest and became a certified teacher. As I endeavoured to heal myself naturally, I began curating a lifestyle that centred yoga/meditation, acupuncture, reiki healing and plant medicine. For seven years I managed the symptoms and slowed the growth of the tumours. When I eventually opted for surgical removal, I learned much about the western medical industrial complex and the challenge of advocating for oneself as a Black woman. I treated my post-surgery healing like a mindfulness practice. Observing, Acknowledging, Accepting and Modifying as needed (OAAM is a concept I bring into my classes now). I learned so much, and I really wanted to offer what I learned to other women who were suffering with uterine dis-ease.

In 2015, I created the Haji Yoga Healing Salon as a Fibroid Support Group for women. As it grew and evolved as a pop-up over that year, the vision broadened, and I realized *all* people could benefit from guidance and support around the creation of a healing lifestyle. In 2016, I shortened the name to Haji Healing Salon and began hosting yoga and acupuncture from my home. In 2018, I opened the first brick and mortar space, offering $10 yoga classes and $25 acupuncture, along with reiki, Asian-style bodywork and sound healing. Black/POC folks came in droves. When Covid hit, we closed and switched to an entirely virtual model, with 25 classes each week. In May of 2021 we completed a build-out of a brand-new space and opened the new Haji Healing Salon and Herbal/Botanical Apothecary. Whew! It's been a journey! Life, love, pain, suffering, and a desire to be liberated from suffering, have all been catalysts for the rise of this enterprise.

What are Haji Healing Salon's core values?

- ❧ AUTHENTICITY: We share our authentic practices, and we *live* what we teach.
- ❧ COURAGE: Healing in a society that thrives on sickness, requires us to have the courage to be *counter-cultural*.
- ❧ COMMUNITY: We are more successful at staying on the path when we are witnessed in our healing and expansion *and* supported as we continue.
- ❧ LOVE: Love energy is the most powerful healing energy there is. All that we do is backed by and rooted in Love.
- ❧ RESPONSIBILITY: We take responsibility for ourselves, for our causes and their effects. We understand we have a responsibility as humans to evolve and we understand how this knowing and the action it inspires, supports the evolution of the collective.
- ❧ SERVICE: Service is one of our responsibilities. As we evolve, we come to understand how best to use our unique gifts to be of service to our communities and the world.

How important has working with/in the local community been to the success of Haji Healing Salon?
A big part of Haji's mission is to inspire and support local healers by providing space for practice, refinement and relationship building. In our five (official) years in business we have employed over 50 healers, teachers and mystics from the southside of Chicago and surrounding areas. We have also thrived because of community partner relationships that have been mutually beneficial. Sometimes that looked like offering our space for a partner programme or sending healers out to co-create with partner organizations; we have also provided healing space for our community of local activists and social justice organizations. We have never paid for advertising but have grown consistently because of the generosity of our clients who consistently share the benefits of being part of Haji with their communities.

Further, I hold strong convictions around the importance of investing in Black/brown communities with a history of disinvestment. My goal with this enterprise has been to lower the barriers that exist for Black people to access these life-enhancing healing modalities. When I think about historical barriers, it's of course been about costs and also location. At our first location, we had a doorbell and buzzer system. After about six months in the space, I realized that this too was a barrier. I started propping the door open, because a closed and locked door might feel like a barrier to some. More people started coming in, and it became a whole different vibe. I think this was a turning point that led to more locals starting to come into the space.

What has been the biggest challenge for your business?
When we first started out the biggest challenge was having a consistent (safe and suitable) space to offer classes and services. After popping up all over the city, it was a relief to finally have a space to call our own. Unfortunately, the storefront we could afford came with lots of issues that wound up being insurmountable. Just a few days after moving into the space, I witnessed a community violence incident just ten feet from where I was standing. It was in the alley right outside of my window. Chaos ensued outside, and this was the day before my opening. Going in, I knew it was a risk to choose that location, and I knew it was an experiment. It was an experiment on a lot of levels. I

had a lot of questions, like: would this kind of business thrive in this neighbourhood and would the community support it to the extent that is required for it to stay open? Are members of the community really going to pay for these types of classes and treatments?

At our first location, it took at least a year of being there to have people who lived right at that intersection in the neighbourhood start coming and accessing our services. Judging by some of the comments I heard later, I think there was an assumption by many of the locals that HHS was another form of gentrification led by white people. It took a while for the locals to realize that the Black woman entering and exiting the building daily is actually the owner.

We were able to build an oasis in a frenetic environment. Something I heard over and over again was that people felt like when they crossed the threshold, they stepped into a whole new world. I have an art and design background, and it is important for me to bring beauty into everything that I do. I knew I wanted to create a beautiful space for Black people to come into and enjoy these practices. The first thing I did was paint the storefront white. I designed window seats that my dad, who is a carpenter, built. The window seats had planters built in, so that I could put the plants directly in them. I had a vision that I wanted people to be able to relax at the window between classes. People naturally congregated there. It was a bench with a high back, and the plants were at the top. The bench served a few purposes. It gave us a little privacy at the window. More importantly, though, the seat backs were hollow. I wanted them to be hollow, so that I could fill them with sandbags, so that if a stray bullet came through the window, it would be stopped before hitting anyone. It was incognito, and I didn't have to make guests worry about the extra measures I was taking to ensure their safety.

We experienced a separate community violence incident right before the start of a yoga class. Nineteen of the 20 registered students still came despite what was happening outside with police and bystanders. That was an extremely powerful Yoga class. Everything about that class – every breath we took, every posture – it was all the ultimate act of resistance. It's like we were saying we will not be stopped by this madness. We will continue to show up and find our peace. We know that this is trickling out, that this is not just for us as individuals.

This is being felt all across 79th Street – the sage, the frankincense, our smiling faces as we leave. Everything is helping to transform this experience. It's so important that we continue.

The additional internal challenges to the space (constant flooding due to faulty plumbing and neighbour negligence) caused frequent interruption to programming with unexpected closures. At the same time, the low rate of rent made it possible for me to save enough money to eventually move to a better space and build it to suit us without the need for loans or crowdfunding. I'm so grateful for that beginning. It was epic. Now that we have a solid space in a new neighbourhood, it seems the new challenge is figuring out the best channels for marketing to new clientele.

Why do you feel like spaces such as Haji Healing Salon are important for the yoga and wellness industry?
Spaces like Haji Healing Salon are important because more mission-driven, heart-centred wellness models are needed. With wellness trending, you find lots of folks jumping into the business for the potential profit. Many wellness businesses are run by folks who are not living the lifestyle they promote – and that can be felt. One thing that makes HHS different is we are unapologetically spiritual. We honour and acknowledge our Source, Ancestors and Spirit Guides in nearly every practice we offer. Authenticity is everything. We also hold space in a way that supports the building of true community. I have frequented so many yoga classes and circles where I left and didn't meet anyone new or didn't feel any sense of connection with anyone beyond the teacher – and sometimes even that opportunity for connectivity was missed. After so many years of being invisibilized as a student and a teacher, I created a business where folks are sure to be seen, heard and felt. We need more of this.

How do diversity, equity and inclusion fit into your business model?
Diversity, equity and inclusion come naturally for me. As someone who grew up within a very diverse spiritual community, I have always felt most comfortable within environments that were rich with multiplicities. While I understand why we are laser-focused on DEI as a nation right now, I doubt we will get to a true sense of what

we are working toward by forcing. Folks will do what is required within companies, institutions and organizations (through diversity hires etc.) but still fail to honour and value one another because of the resentment that backs being forced to change. I and those I am in community with – artists, healers, mystics, misfits – *are* diversity; we *uplift* equity and we *live* inclusive lives by valuing all the ways life shows up. Within HHS, we have historically prioritized POC folks for hiring, but ultimately, we hire those who have the most integrity, authenticity and efficacy in their practice. Elders, LGBTQ+, disabled, gender and racially diverse communities have been represented in Haji's client and practitioner base from the beginning . . . naturally.

Where do you see the business in the next three to five years?
In three to five years, Haji Healing Salon continues to thrive as a vibrant social wellness enterprise that inspires and supports the creation of a healing lifestyle for people everywhere. Our hybrid model provides in-person and virtual wellness, and our community has expanded to include a strong base of wellness curators who own and operate our multiple locations across the country. Haji Healing Salon is an innovator in health and wellness, inspiring folks all over the world to make healing a lifestyle and thriving resistance!

Interview with HealHaus
Below is a transcribed interview with Elisa Schankle, co-founder of HealHaus.[16] HealHaus is based in Brooklyn, New York in the United States. It is an inclusive space focused on holistic health and wellness.

What was the catalyst for opening HealHaus?
The catalyst was a lot of people's stories – specifically people of colour. We opened almost four years ago, and it's weird to think we've been virtual now for almost half that time.

Before that, in my early twenties, I was dealing with anxiety and depression, and I was working in a corporate environment. I wasn't happy. I ended up discovering therapy, which really helped me to understand and unpack a lot of my family trauma. I also met with a naturopathic doctor and really got into how to heal myself naturally – and how these things can be managed. It's really just about understanding Earth medicine, holistic medicine. I got into different diet alternatives, and herbal medicine. And that kind of led me down the path into my twenties and my thirties.

It became integrated into my lifestyle, and I knew it was something I wanted to share with my community and so I started with sharing it with family members. It was very simple. Like with my grandmother, who had high blood pressure, or with a cousin of mine who was dealing with fibromyalgia, and helping them with anti-inflammatory remedies. Mindfulness was always a daily part of my practice. I got energy attuned. All these things that I was doing – I was confused and perplexed as to why they weren't accessible to my community. I knew that was going to become a part of my path at some point.

And so I met Darien, my co-founder. We were both on transformational journeys and had known each other for ten years. It just kind of became this integrated thing where we started talking about what if there was a space for body, mind and spirit that addressed all aspects of our being and all aspects of our healing, because it's not just one thing. So within making this space, it was about reflecting not only on the practice or the client, but also the practitioner. And understanding that in order for inclusivity to be holistic or come full circle, you have to see yourself reflected. And then you have to also see the person next to you being reflective.

What are HealHaus's core values?
It's interesting, I've never thought about it in a list format. I've never consciously been like, "these are our core values". I feel like my brain doesn't really work that way. I kind of just live what I preach.

It's definitely inclusivity. It's accessibility. It's transparency. For practitioners to be able to be who they are and offer their greatest offering and for that to resonate with whoever is receiving it. We're not about making this packaging up pretty, but we're also about being ourselves and having fun with it. It's a combination. I'd definitely say HealHaus is integrity driven.

We're really big on the work that we do, the type of work that we do and its quality. I would say the quality and also the source of where that's coming from. We're really big on whoever is facilitating something, that they're experts in that, and that even more importantly, maybe it comes from their lineage or their practices. Ancestral resonance is really important to me. And therefore I think that is reflected in HealHaus.

There are more core values. Community is everything. We don't run without our community of practitioners and the community that attends classes. We move like a family. I'm friends with all of our practitioners. Some of them are very close friends of mine. And that's how we started. We started out with our network and then branched out. Everyone kind of moves like a family with us and for us. It works. So that's definitely something. We're very family oriented.

How important has working with and in the local community been to the success of HealHaus?
I haven't been asked questions like this in a long time, and I feel like it's making me almost emotional because we've been [physically] closed for two years. We're finally going to reopen in March 2022. We tried to reopen in August last year. With New York City and the mandates, it was just too much.

I've been missing the in-person space so much. And our local community is the beginning of how we even started and the core of what we do – being in Bed-Stuy[17] and just seeing people from the community, specifically Black people who have never, ever done any of these classes before, or have never tried something that's in our café, or been to therapy or any of these things. Being able to have that access to that space, whether it's a PE class or donation class, which we would do weekly where people could just give what they have. It's so integral and crucial to what we do and what we stand for, even though we're moving into the digital space. In-person space is so important to us, because it's really how you feel the vibration of this work. Our Brooklyn community, Brooklyn itself, is definitely the underbelly of who we are and what we do. A lot of our practitioners, who started out with us and live in Brooklyn, are still in the virtual community. Some of them are still going to be in the in-person community. It's very important.

What has been the biggest challenge for your business?
There've been many challenges in different phases. I'd say the biggest challenge is right now, which I can only describe as pivoting [due to

the pandemic]. But honestly, the pivot is what has taken our business to the next level.

As far as a challenge turning into a blessing, it's meant being able to move online faster than we thought we were going to be able to do and to start reaching a global community – which has been really incredible, because for us, it's about how do we reach everyone? Especially people of colour globally to have access to this work. That was something that started out as a challenge. But the bigger challenge right now is resources.

It's about being a startup, being an entrepreneur and wanting to expand and grow. And the reality is just being able to get funding, in general, is super hard. I think for Black women, it's that 0.0 per cent of Black women get funding in the venture capital space. Just maintaining my faith and my grounded-ness of what's going to happen, but still dealing with the realities of me and my partner running five aspects of our business is hard. It's hard too because I want to be able to be in a position where I can hire senior leaders so that I can delegate more than I am right now. I definitely say the biggest challenge is funding to be able to resource and expand and grow the way that I want to, and the way that I want to support not only the clients but practitioners in this journey.

Why do you feel like spaces such as HealHaus are important for the yoga and wellness industry?
It's about representation. A person of colour often doesn't feel safe in regular, white-dominated wellness spaces. I don't even attend them. I get invited to things, or I have access to them, but because it just doesn't resonate with me any time I've been in those spaces [I don't go]. I've been harmed, whether that's passively or directly. And it's just a position that I don't want to put myself in. I think a lot of people of colour feel like me in that they don't feel safe. And when you're in a space where your mental health is involved, your wellbeing is involved, you really don't want to put that in the hands of someone that maybe you're risking your not being received or seen or felt. That's why it's so important for practitioners who are Black and brown to be hired and to be supported financially. In doing the work, they need to feel

compensated and supported. It follows that then clients come to that space, that base, and they feel seen. It comes full circle. You need to see the reflection on both ends and people of colour need to be supported in general, whether that's financially, mentally, emotionally. It's just very important.

How do diversity, equity and inclusion fit into your business model?
It's very natural for us. I don't harp on being a Black-owned business or equity inclusion because honestly, it's something I don't understand that people wouldn't even do naturally. For me, it is just a natural reflection of my community and how I move. I think everyone should be integrating that naturally into their business structure, into their hiring process, into everything – like who they're catering to, what their products are like and so forth.

It's literally like breathing air. Why would you not do something that reflects the collective? I'm very big on stressing the importance of if that's not something that comes naturally to you, you need to do the work to where that flows naturally within you and your organization.

Where do you see the business in the next three to five years?
In the next three to five years, we will have a HealHaus app. The HealHaus app will be launched next year, possibly spring.

The next two to five years will see us really dominating the virtual wellness space and having a network of community members that are worldwide and tapping into practitioners that are worldwide and being able to support people near and far.

It's about changing the narrative of what wellness looks like and who it's for on a mass level. I know we've already gained notoriety of really being the blueprint around that and having such a vast range of offerings, and so for us, it's just being able to build on-demand content and our physical space. I would love to see a physical space in LA. I have always said if we had one other physical location, that would be it.

Working with Our Emotions

In this chapter, we have addressed the pivotal role of studio owners in creating equitable and inclusive environments in which people of all social identities and backgrounds feel welcome and *safe enough* to practise.[18] I have also offered examples of studios that are owned by people creating their own models to serve communities that have been historically underrepresented and underserved in the wellness space.

The details of this chapter may elicit conflicting emotions in its readers. For some readers, it may feel like an unachievable and impossible task to create spaces that are truly representative of wider parts of society. I invite you to refer back to the step-by-step guide to get you started. It is not a task to be completed in a day or even a year. Hell, it's not even a task. It's a different or new-to-you approach to working. For other readers, the chapter may feel too business-like. This is a conflict I have encountered often in my consulting practice. Business owners in the wellness space are, nevertheless, business owners. Leadership teams often consist of people with business or commercial backgrounds across the usual disciplines, such as law or consulting, as well as at least one owner/founder who has been emotionally or spiritually touched by some practice, whether Yoga, somatics, martial arts, a combination of these or something else entirely. These are also not mutually exclusive; in many cases this is the same person. The business or commercial side recognizes the driving force of financial performance. Without sales, revenue and profit, the studio or business will not survive. Facts. However, the patrons are not concerned with the money, and in many cases, they have unrealistic assumptions about how much a wellness space or yoga studio (or chain) earns. Their expectations have everything to do with how they are made to feel in the space. As a studio owner and/or manager, you must be able to hold both of these truths side by side. This chapter is not asking you to reimagine your business model. That would take a whole book rather than a chapter. It is, however, guiding you through tried-and-tested steps of a holistic approach to more equitable and inclusive wellness spaces.

In the following, a practice is offered that will support you in working with your emotions, even or especially when you are in a reactive state. Developing a wise relationship to our emotions – even when they are conflicted, underdeveloped or conditioned – is a fundamental piece of self-work that will prove urgently important on the path to equity and inclusion.

Practice Break: RAIN

Let us move into the practice. You can practise on your own or in a group.

Start by coming into a seated posture that feels comfortable to you. If you choose to sit in a chair or on your sofa, bring your feet firmly to the ground. Have the feet slightly apart so that the hips can relax. If your feet do not touch the ground, place a pillow or folded blanket beneath them to bring the floor to you. If you choose to sit on the floor, use a cushion so that the knees are able to relax toward the floor. Your palms, placed comfortably on your thighs, can face upward for opening or downward for grounding.

Allow your body to settle. Notice if you need any final adjustments before coming into stillness.

Soften the gaze or close your eyes, depending on your environment and how you are currently feeling. It is not necessary to have the eyes completely closed. If you are feeling tired or sleepy, you may want to keep your eyes slightly open.

Bring your awareness to your breath, as an anchor for attention. Do not try to control or alter the breath. Simply allow yourself to rest in the awareness of your breath. If your breath is not available to you in this moment, bring your awareness to your connection to the ground.

After some time, open your awareness to the sensations of the body. Tune in to the sensory experience, beginning at the feet and travelling up through to the crown of the head and back down again.

After some time, further open your awareness to the sounds around you. If this becomes too much or too distracting, reduce your field of awareness to the sensations within the body.

Once you are feeling settled, begin to observe how emotions come and go.

Notice where you feel any given emotion in your body. Rest your awareness there momentarily – without judgement – before allowing your awareness to again move through the body.

Without the use of force, notice subtler states in the body as well, such as tension or openness.

Now call forth an event or incident that you would like to explore that is not too triggering or traumatizing.

R – Recognize the emotions that are present for you once you have the event front of mind. Take some time for this without getting lost in reliving the event.

A – Allow the exploration with curiosity and inquisitiveness. Remain here for a while.

I – Investigate the thoughts and emotions surrounding the experience with kindness and compassion. Where do you feel the emotion(s) in your body? What is your reaction or response to the emotion(s)? How has your attitude shifted? Remain here for a while.

N – Nurture with compassion without attaching to the thoughts or emotions. Ask yourself what you are feeling as you continue to explore. Offer yourself kindness and compassion without the baggage of self-pity or judgement – of things being either good or bad (a state of non-judgement). And remember that nothing is personal (impersonal).

At your own pace, begin to bring your awareness back into the space. You may want to first rotate your wrists and stretch your arms.

Take a few deeper, more intentional breaths.

In your own time, open your eyes or raise your gaze.

CHAPTER 7

TEACHER TRAINING SCHOOLS: STOP THE CHURN AND HOLD YOURSELVES TO A HIGHER STANDARD

In chapter 3, I addressed some of the elemental issues pertaining to the curricula taught at most teacher training schools. I noted that there are over 7,000 Registered Yoga Schools (RYS) through US-based Yoga Alliance, the largest non-profit association representing the yoga community. Between January and June of 2020, the British Wheel of Yoga (BWY), the United Kingdom's largest yoga membership organization, offered at least eight teacher trainings. And there are hundreds more schools that regularly train teachers and, for their own reasons, are not represented through Yoga Alliance or BWY.

I invited teachers to reflect on the following questions in chapter 3: How did 200 hours become the norm? Is this an arbitrary number or does it have meaning?

- ♣ How was the core curriculum of your teacher training crafted? Why is the physical practice emphasized above all other limbs?
- ♣ To what extent were wisdom seat holders of South Asian heritage centred in the process of creating the two largest governing bodies? Why is that?
- ♣ How does a western credentialing system serve a South Asian wisdom tradition?

If you are a yoga teacher training school owner or manager, I would encourage you to read chapter 3 before continuing with this chapter, as it will offer you the opportunity to reflect on your choices as a teacher before focusing on your role as a teacher trainer.

In this chapter, we first turn our attention to the economics of teacher training schools. I understand that many yoga teachers, studio and teacher training school owners have an image of themselves that is far from driven by money. But let's be real. There is no survival in today's world as teachers or business owners without money. From my consulting practice, I know that financial realities drive most, if not all, decisions around how many courses to offer on what subjects and at what price. This was true before the global Covid-19 pandemic and has been amplified throughout it.

The basic approach is known as the minimum principle in economics. In reference to training schools, it can be understood as training as many people as possible in the shortest amount of time possible (typically 30 days/one month) given the set of standards and requirements by the accreditation bodies. If you were to go to your search engine of choice and search yoga teacher trainings, you would reliably find a significant number of results pointing you to trainings in beautiful locations across South and Southeast Asia, or Central and South America, making training experiences comparable to a month-long holiday in an *exotic* location. You might expect that this will have changed due to the ongoing consequences of the global Covid-19 pandemic; however, the opposite has been the case. With Yoga Alliance relaxing its requirements around in-person trainings, many schools have been able to maintain or even increase their offerings now that they are able to do so both virtually, pre-recorded and in-person. Let's peel back the layers.

Steal a Little, Steal a Lot – Asteya in Practice

Teacher training schools, as all other businesses, have financial obligations. Some of these include venue (whether rented or owned), teaching staff, administrative staff, domain and web hosting, online tools, such as online course platforms, accreditation and subscription fees, marketing, and more. Depending on school location, these fees can quickly add up. At the same time, schools in North America and Europe tend to recoup their costs per training after the first three to, at most, five students have enrolled. Schools based in South and Southeast Asia do so after the first two to, at most, four students have enrolled.

JOURNALING PROMPTS

» What is my motivation in training yoga teachers?

» What is my motivation in actively participating in the business of training yoga teachers?

» To what extent do I see my business model represented in the economic minimum principle?

» To what extent do Yogic principles and values, as outlined in the *Yoga Sutras*, align with my school's business model, values, mission and purpose?

» How would I earn a living if I did not own a school?

In chapter 2, I discussed the meaning of asteya and asked readers to consider the less obvious forms of stealing, such as colonialist regimes depriving Indigenous populations access to and use of their first tongue, culture and wisdom traditions. If you own and/or run a teacher training school based in a continent or region that you or your family do not originate from, you are invited to reflect on the following questions:

» What is your motivation for locating your school in a region to which you have no familial ties?

» How would you describe your fluency in the Indigenous languages common in the area?

» Is your teaching faculty representative of the local population? Why is that?

» Does your teaching faculty include people of South Asian heritage? Why is that?

» Where do your trainees commonly hail from? Is your teaching faculty representative of that composition? Why is that?

IN REAL LIFE

Learning Sanskrit

Yoga Journal offers a course on learning Sanskrit (off to a good start!) called "Sanskrit 101: A Beginner's Guide". This introductory course is taught by Richard Rosen (and now we're back to business as usual). Richard Rosen is a white American man, who began his yoga teaching journey in the 1980s. He has written several yoga books and has reviewed even more. My critique here is not the usual patriarchal-colonized challenge of his qualifications. I have never studied with him. I also have no reason to question his skills or expertise. The issue is that *Yoga Journal* chose to keep it basic (a pattern pointed out in chapter 2) by having one of its white American contributing editors teach a course that could and should be taught by a South Asian scholar. Sanskrit is a classical language of South Asia, in which most of the Yogic texts that we refer to and teach today were written. Sanskrit is the sacred language of Yoga. One of many ways to appreciate rather than appropriate is for an organization such as *Yoga Journal* to ensure that all its Sanskrit courses are led by South Asian scholars.

BWY Certificate Course

Paul Fox, former chair of BWY in the UK, prioritized modernizing the membership organization during his tenure. One of his priorities was creating different pathways for underrepresented member groups to become certified teachers (see chapter 3 for questions on decolonizing credentialing) and/or join as members. From 2017 to 2019, a BWYQ certificate course was designed and offered specifically for Black women and women of colour. It was the first course of its kind in BWY's 52-year history. As Fox is a white British man, he invited Jaz Mullings-Lambert, a Black British woman and BWY regional lead of North London at the time, and myself, who at the time had no affiliation with BWY, to join him on the course as co-tutors.

The course was offered at a subsidized fee, and all the tutors took a reduced fee to make this possible. Trainees could also create a two-year payment plan to pay their course fees over time. The course was offered on one Saturday per month, rather than all at once, which made it possible for full-time employed women (many of whom were mothers and/or caretakers) to participate and also allowed trainees to deepen their practice if they did not meet the usual prerequisite experience required on other courses that completed in a matter of months. Fox also sought to create a new pathway to becoming a Diploma Course Tutor (DCT),[19] so that BWY would formally recognize the time and work invested by the two Black female tutors, who also acted as mentors to the trainees during the course. Because at the time there were no Black DCTs, this would have also made it possible to offer future courses without the need for a white DCT. Most of the changes Fox tried to integrate were met with great opposition and ultimately were not pursued further at the end of his tenure. After the social justice protests that took place in the summer of 2020, the BWY leadership team did take some minimal actions to begin work on a DEI strategy. Most of those actions were based on recommendations made by some of the graduates of this course.

What Now?

Some of you may be reading this chapter and feeling attacked. The grumbles may sound like, "Are you saying I should stop teaching yoga?" Or, "So white people shouldn't teach at all?" Or even, "You aren't even South Asian, and my South Asian friend said that they think it's great that I teach!" I am not suggesting that readers should generally not be teaching or training teachers, though there is a discussion to be had about one's ability to *teach* Yoga (see chapter 11). Perhaps you are feeling quite receptive to what you have read. Either way, I invite you to continue onto the next section for some implementable actions to help you align your Yogic values with your business actions.

Things You Can Change Immediately

Curriculum:
- ✤ Assess the course content with an equity and inclusion lens.
- ✤ Create more space for content outside of the subjects of āsana, anatomy and physiology.

❧ Ensure that your curriculum includes the subject of power dynamics in teaching practice, racial hierarchy and positionality, as well as consent.

❧ Ensure your curriculum includes content on teaching to the specific needs of different populations of people.

Teaching Staff:

❧ Diversify your teaching faculty.

❧ Ensure that people of South Asian heritage are on the faculty – more than one! (No tokenizing, please.)

❧ Ensure that people of marginalized social identities are teaching subjects such as power dynamics, intersectionality, consent, etc.

Trainee Population:

❧ Send surveys to all participants of every course.

❧ Try to reach a feedback rate of at least 80 per cent.

❧ Hire experts who can complete an audit of your website, social media channels, etc. to ascertain what populations are being overlooked.

❧ Integrate flexibility into your courses, such as payment plans, scholarships, dates and times, etc.

Business Model:

❧ Consider creating a sliding scale for tuition.

❧ Make payment plans the norm.

Radical Darshan

After George Floyd's murder, yoga teacher and mentor Jonelle Lewis hosted several Instagram Live events. One session was with Kallie Schut on 11 June 2020. It was entitled "Cultural Appropriation in Yoga and Wellness". Together, Jonelle and Kallie highlighted specific areas where appropriation most commonly shows up in yoga, and Kallie offered ways to honour Yoga and its roots without appropriating the wisdom tradition. One session was with me on 18 June 2020. It was entitled "Belonging and Inclusion in Wellness". During that conversation, we scratched the surface on the topics covered in chapter 6. The sessions ended with Leila Sadeghee on 25 June 2020. The final conversation in that series was entitled "Tools to Dismantle Racism". Leila and Jonelle addressed yoga teachers and solopreneurs to provide resources on how to do the work of dismantling racism, and other forms of oppression, in their teaching practice.

With the feedback Jonelle received from the series, she decided to approach Kallie, Leila and me about founding a yoga teacher training school. Leila had been delivering a 200-hour training for nearly eight years at the time. Kallie had begun offering ten-hour courses to yoga teachers and other wellness practitioners on cultural appropriation. Similarly, I was offering six-hour immersions for yoga teachers on racial and intersectional equity. The group of four came together to create Radical Darshan, a 300-hour advanced yoga teacher training school.

One of the first major decisions we made as founders and lead trainers was on accreditation. Initially, we did not want to seek Yoga Alliance accreditation for the school for many of the reasons that are discussed here and in chapter 3. However, we eventually made the decision to have the school accredited. Firstly, there are next to no schools offering the number of hours and quality of content on the subject of antiracism and colonialism that Radical Darshan does. We also knew that our yoga school would especially appeal to Black teachers and teachers of colour. Thus, it was important to us that people who choose to complete our trainings are recognized for their commitment to social justice and intersectional equity and can pursue every opportunity available to them. The process of becoming accredited was not without its challenges, but we persevered. We will continuously assess if the accreditation is necessary, but we feel strongly about ensuring that folks doing anti-oppression work in Yoga and wellness – especially Black, Indigenous and People of Colour, whose credentials are scrutinized and called into question more than those of their white counterparts – are recognized for a training with both a great time and self-work investment.

We call Radical Darshan a gift of collective freedom. Our teaching faculty is majority South Asian heritage. Further, the teaching faculty identify as women, non-binary and trans. Our ethos is drawn from our collective work in Yoga, antiracism and social justice. Our teachings are inspired by deeper readings of the *Bhagavadgītā* and Patañjali's *Yoga Sutras*, which draw out equity, inclusion and justice principles, as well as a collective commitment to liberation.

We actively invite and welcome teachers ready to take a bold step forward which entails risk and courage through heterodoxical thinking and decolonized patterns of behaviour. Those steps manifest as:

✿   taking responsibility and being held to account for what and how you teach;

✿   moving beyond boundaries of conventional power dynamics;

✿   adopting a liberatory critical teaching approach;

✿   integrating and embodying justice and equity in teaching spaces;

✿   creatively building anti-oppressive and pro-unity relationships with students;

✿   growing and applying the principles of inclusion and compassionate collective care.

We do not claim to have all the answers or to get everything right. We are, however, committed to our own (un-)learning journeys and supporting others in the process. Our model is just one way of decolonizing Yoga.

Moving through Fear

This chapter has offered a lot of space for reflecting through journaling and real-life examples of what doing things another way could look like for teacher training schools. The chapter also includes tactical changes any school can make almost immediately to change how practitioners become teachers.

A great obstacle to change is fear of the unfamiliar. When faced with two options, people will often choose the familiar one, even if they don't like it, because it is the option they know. In human history, many moments of social uprising have come after the familiar has simply become too unbearable. Whether we, too, now find ourselves at a tipping point, is for the astrologers and historians to decide. We can, however, ignite our inner fire for change through breath work. The lower abdomen is an area that, across Eastern traditions, is related to power, creativity and self-knowing.

Kapālabhāti prāṇāyāma, or kriyā, is a great practice to create heat in the part of the body that connects to our creativity and power. *Kapāla* means "skull" and *bhāti* means "light". The practice focuses on a vigorous exhalation and passive inhalation, with retention lasting less than a second in between. Do not practise when menstruating heavily or pregnant. If at any time you become unsettled, simply discontinue the breathing practice, and come back to long, deep breaths.

Practice Break: Kapālabhāti Prāṇāyāma

Let's move into the practice.

Sit in any comfortable position.

Place your hands on your thighs, palms facing upward.

Exhale fully the breath in the lungs.

Inhale normally to begin and expel the breath with a quick and forceful blast. Repeat.

Do four to eight rounds of these inhalations and exhalations (or, for experienced practitioners, for 30 seconds) to complete one cycle.

Then inhale deeply. Pause at the top of breath and engage mūla bandha (lift the pelvic floor or cervical mouth). After 10 to 15 seconds, exhale slowly and deeply.

Repeat these cycles three or four times.

End in śavāsana.

Over time you can extend your cycles or increase the number of cycles.

CHAPTER 8

BRANDS: YOUR CONSUMERS DEMAND AND DESERVE BETTER

While the terms "brand" and "company" are often used interchangeably, they are different. A brand is an intangible asset that helps consumers identify a company and its products. With the proliferation of the Internet, social media and smart phones, the relationship between brands and consumers has radically shifted. Similar to the education system described in chapter 5, it used to be that the role of companies was to tell consumers what to eat, how to dress, and how to live. If you wanted to cook for convenience, there were food and beverage brands for that. If you wanted to present as a professional in the workplace, there were retail brands for that. If you wanted to impress on wheels, there were automotive brands for that too.

Today, the relationship between brands and consumers is much less directive and much more participative. Through technological adaptations, such as computer cookies, brands have tried to become better listeners (or, rather, lurkers). As cookies are phased out, brands are being forced to do even more to listen and understand consumer groups better, rather than simply direct their lifestyle choices. Social media influencers, many of whom do not have paid partnerships with brands, offer their two cents to their audiences on brands they love or love to hate. Podcasts and vlogs also have a role to play in flattening the brand-consumer hierarchy, as hobby investigators and journalists present research – with varying degrees of reliability, validity and rigour – to inform their audiences on hot topics related to brands, big and small.

As information has become more accessible, it has meant that companies have been obligated to become more self-aware. Their dubious business practices can no longer be tucked away into the appendices of their annual reports. Companies have had to answer tough questions from governing bodies and consumers alike. It is no coincidence that the business values taught at every prestigious business school around the globe – i.e., that a company's primary goal is to enrich its shareholders/maximize shareholder value – have been called into question over the last few years as collective social consciousness has been raised. Consequently, consumers relate to brands more personally than before.

In some ways, this is good news for brands. The more personal a brand feels to its consumers the better. Brand loyalty and brand passion thrive on the positive personal experiences of its consumers. The deeper brand loyalty is, the higher the profitability of the brand. The personal relationship consumers nurture with brands also means that consumers treat brands as an extension of themselves. And that's where things get tricky. If we turn our attention specifically to the yoga industry, then we may find ourselves trying to drive down a mountain in a two-wheel-drive vehicle while it's raining in below-freezing temperatures – slippery!

Brands, and the companies behind them, demonstrated how unprepared they were to rise to the occasion of the largest show of organized civil unrest in over five decades after George Floyd's murder. Some responded immediately (great!) without the humility required to acknowledge their own history of discrimination (nope!). Some only responded after several days as they waited to see in which direction the wind was blowing (we see you). Again, others responded with actions that were unimaginative, disingenuous and thoughtless, in some cases even offensive. Consumers were having none of it.

If you are a brand or marketing professional, you may be thinking that, at this point, you can't win for losing. But that's not what I am saying. Instead, brands should:

♣   create clarity around their values and the purpose of their action;

♣   align the action to reflect historical activity and learnings from missteps;

♣   grow (brand) equity in communities through long-term commitment.

JOURNALING PROMPTS

»   To what extent have you done research on public views concerning major political and social matters that affect your audiences and society at large?

»   To what extent have you done research on how consumers view your company's or brand's historical actions and values?

»   What work is your company doing to build brand and social equity in the communities in which it resides?

»   What are the priorities of senior leadership concerning equity and inclusion, and how are these priorities reflected in every aspect of the business – from supplier diversity through to the marketing and advertising process?

Spotify releases an annual research report, Culture Next, in partnership with Archrival (2021) as well as Culture Co-op, b3 Intelligence and Lucid (2020), to gain insights into how Millennials and Gen Zs relate to brands. In the 2020 publication, 93 per cent of Gen Zs surveyed chose "purpose" over "politics" when examining what they want to see out of brands. Eighty-three per cent of US respondents recognized the Black Lives Matter movement of 2020 as a "cultural wake-up call". And that wake-up call directly influenced their behaviour, leading them to actively turn to Black-hosted podcasts for education and Black-music playlists to support Black-owned businesses.

In the research published in 2021, Spotify found that 39 per cent of Millennials and 42 per cent of Gen Zs in the UK believe listening to music without the background knowledge of the culture it came from is problematic. This points to a greater desire of young people to participate in culture, connect with like-minded communities, and use cultural entertainment such as music and podcasts to educate themselves about other cultures. The research also identified that these groups do not identify with the gender norms of winters past. Women-identified folks have more range than many brands allow room for. These insights are transferable to the yoga and wellness industry.

Clearly Aligned Values and Action

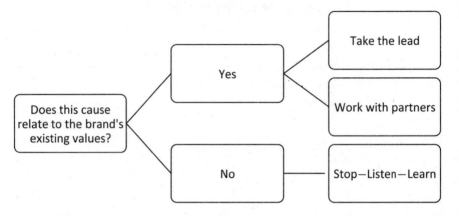

Above: A decision tree for brands when making the first decision on taking public action for a specific cause.

Authenticity, an overused yet hard-to-define word, plays an important role in times of social crisis and political turmoil. Over the last few years, we can observe how consumers judge brands through punishment and reward, depending on how authentic they are perceived to be. Some company executives complain that it is not their role to respond to every social cause that takes over the 24-hour news cycle on any given day. I would counter that it is not necessary to respond every time if the company is already known to be doing the work. However, there are events that call for executives and brands to speak up, loudly and clearly.

If the event or circumstance does not relate to the brand's existing values, it is best to take a seat. To help consumers understand that decision, brands should speak up about what they are doing to educate themselves now. It's never too late. The process of education has to be a sincere one. It cannot be an out, in place of taking action. Brands must keep their consumers informed about the journey and, where appropriate, let the journey be a participative one where consumers can come along too.

If the cause does relate to the brand's existing values, the next consideration is to decide if the brand should take the lead or work with partners. If the brand is already recognized as a thought leader on the subject, then it is likely well positioned to take the lead. If the cause lies firmly outside of the brand's expertise, then the brand should work with partners such as grassroots organizations, influencers who have been doing the work, or even other brands, companies and startups, which are the experts, to deliver an action that is purposeful with measurable impact.

Avoid Revisionist History

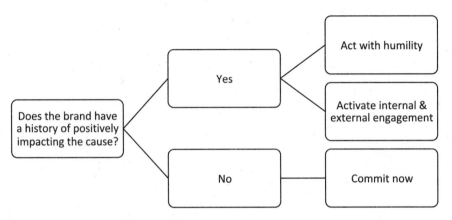

Above: A decision tree to help brands decide what actions to take – either internally or externally focused – in the case of a social crisis.

Senior executives will be tempted to want to profit, in the realest sense of the word, from any social actions taken. Large corporations, of course, have dedicated policies to pro bono work. However, there is something different about a moment of social or political crisis. As we have witnessed time and again, the consumer backlash is usually swift and severe. The goal of action is not to profit or to gain new consumers. Instead, it is to act meaningfully and in a way that may positively impact people negatively affected in an emergency.

If the brand does not have a history of leading change in that particular area or has a history of doing the opposite in a related area, then this is not the time to take externally targeted action. Instead, the brand needs to commit publicly to the internally focused steps it is going to take to do better going forward. The public commitment should include an acknowledgment of, and apology for, historical failures and oversights, as well as a clear outline of next steps, timeline and budget.

If the brand has a history of delivering meaningful and measurably impactful work related to the cause at hand, then the brand should take action with humility. That action can be communicated without boasting and can be shared without being promoted. Further, the brand should look to lead actions that activate internal engagement within the organization, as well as external engagement through those channels that are appropriate and available to it.

Build Community and Advance Equity

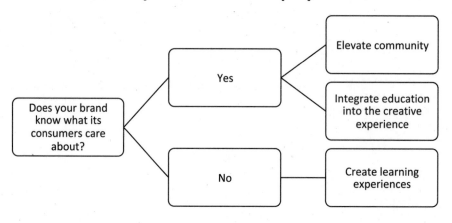

Above: A decision tree for brands, highlighting steps to advancing equity through creativity.

In seeking sustainable change and aspiring to a world absent of an oppressive dominant culture, brands have to use their social good will and financial power to build community. If a brand does not know what its consumers care about, then it must first embed learning experiences into its processes to get to know its consumers better. Those processes should be crafted in such a way that the learning is reciprocal and transparent. I recognize that consumers sit on a spectrum of opinions concerning every socio-political issue that the world is faced with today. I acknowledge that the spectrum is not linear. And it has become clear that younger consumers approach culture and difference with more openness and adaptability than present in the Baby Boomer generation. With a focus on learning experiences, there is an opportunity to reach vastly different consumers, because there is no imperative to arrive at a particular destination.

If a brand does know what its consumers care about, then the next step is to elevate communities doing work in those areas. Even in a globalized world, consumers care about the uniqueness and specific needs of micro-communities. Brand partnerships give communities the opportunity to tell their own stories. No one else needs to do this for them. Utilizing the creative minds that continue to move the brand forward to take people on a learning journey is engaging for consumers and exciting for brands. The most important aspect is that brands recognize their role in shaping public opinion and, in acknowledging the great responsibility that comes with that, commit to doing the continuous work of remaining in dialogue with everyday people.

IN REAL LIFE

What Bad Looks Like

Drunk Yoga® (obviously we're off to a hella bad start with this brand name) claims to want to make yoga more accessible by creating interactive yoga experiences. The name alone will alienate people who do not drink alcohol for personal, social or religious reasons irrespective of whether alcohol is being served at every event. I don't buy the accessibility angle. But let's continue. Drunk Yoga® organized and promoted an event that was meant to take place on 31 July 2020. It was stated in the event description that all event proceeds would be donated to the Innocence Project.

The Innocence Project was founded in 1992 by Peter Neufeld and Barry Scheck at Cardoza School of Law. The charity's mission is to free the staggering number of people who remain incarcerated through DNA testing, while reforming the criminal justice system to prevent future injustice. Some of their cases have received a great deal of media attention over the last few years, including the exoneration of two of the men who were convicted of the murder of Malcolm X.

I was shocked to learn that the Innocence Project would allow their name to be used in association with a brand like Drunk Yoga® so I reached out. Within just a few hours, the Innocence Project team responded to my email enquiry, stating that they had not been contacted about the event in advance. The team had not been alerted to the event before my email.

If you can get past the misappropriation of the word Yoga and the harm caused by connecting it to inebriation (I cannot), then you can use the above model to easily identify what went wrong. The brand stands for "fun" corporate events to loosen people up through drinks while going through a vinyasa sequence. No connection to social justice can be found on the website. Even if the founder, or others, felt moved to respond during the social justice protests of the summer of 2020, they could have done so quietly by simply donating to the Innocence Project. Or they could have, at the very minimum, contacted the Innocence Project before using their name on event pages. However, this level of attention and awareness cannot be expected from a brand that has registered such a name in complete disregard for the origins of Yoga.

What Good Looks Like – Interview with Yogamatters

Below is a written interview with Twanna Doherty, Managing Director of Yogamatters, which was conducted in November 2021. Yogamatters was founded in 1996 with the aim of making yoga equipment available and accessible to all.

How do you define Yogamatters's purpose and vision?
Our purpose at Yogamatters is to champion wellbeing for all. To welcome, speak to, encourage and inspire people to find and restore their balance through accessible and sustainable wellbeing products and content.

How does your purpose show up in how you work and the products you offer?
The way we work, as well as the products and content we offer, all stem from our roots as a company. For us, it's key that we are accessible for every type of customer and that we are inclusive in a way that works for them. How we talk to our customers is also very important to us: the way we describe our products, the knowledge we impart, the recognition of where you are on your wellbeing journey. We collaborate with others where we are not the experts and use our established community to build and share experiences.

What has changed for your company since the start of the Covid-19 pandemic?
Before Covid-19 our focus was on sustainability – people and planet. The pandemic accelerated our desire to learn more and "do more".

However, the standout change is the way we worked as a team – by being more agile. Our customers' needs and shopping patterns changed, and we had to adjust to meet their needs. What has changed most is how we connect with, and try to support, our community of practitioners; a change we wholeheartedly embraced. Ultimately, Covid-19 brought us closer to our community. For example, we decided to offer a weekly yoga class free of charge, intended as an offering of practice, a Yogamatters wellbeing gift. Everyone was welcomed whether a customer or not. We had no grand plan; we simply wanted to connect through practice. So, we started working with a local (London-based) yoga teacher who helped us do what we do – reach out and serve the Yoga journey. It made a positive impact on us, and on our community.

Why do you believe that your customers feel good about buying your products?
Yogamatters is a very trusted brand built on ethics and sustainability from its beginnings back in 1996. Our collection of over 2,500 yoga and wellbeing products have been carefully curated from brands and makers that share our values. We put a lot of effort into colour, pattern and aesthetic to deliver a sense of happiness and fulfilment to your practice and environment – creating a true feel-good factor for those using and receiving our products.

What is your team's strategy in responding to major incidents?
Some major incidents simply cannot be planned for, but we have learned never to make rash decisions. Good leadership requires quick but careful consideration. This is not easy but is key and we have to be prepared to get it wrong.

What is something you personally care about that informs your leadership?
Listening, learning and growing. Being curious, open, fair and creating opportunities. Having a clear sense of purpose and creating meaningful connections. Trusting my instincts and encouraging others to do the same. Being grounded.

Doing the Good Work

In this chapter, I have outlined how brands can go about making decisions in critical moments. Those decisions will also inform long-term commitments to change processes within organizations. The decision tree diagrams in this chapter may make the process appear straightforward, but that is only true in an ideal world. There is, unfortunately, much that is not ideal in today's world. Companies are filling the gaps of democratic governments as populism polarizes public discourse around themes of the role of systemic racism and social justice in our everyday lives. Further, the makeup of the executive committees and boards of most large organizations are not known for their diversity. The people who can speak to current matters of social justice, racial and intersectional equity, are underrepresented at the executive level, often do not have access to senior leadership, and/or are not empowered to speak about these issues without fear of repercussions. If you are reading this, what role can and will you play in changing that reality?

The ego, as used in colloquial speech, is often associated with self-centred or selfish behaviour. Such behaviours are typically considered negative. If taking a wider view, the ego – in a Yogic context – is a person's identification with their current human form. The ego represents an attachment to the material world and the physical body. Through Yoga and other practices, it is possible to liberate oneself from that attachment, i.e., to progress from self-centredness to Self-realization.

After achieving a certain level of success in the material world, it can be especially difficult to detach one's identity from one's achievements. The people behind the brands, who have worked to create something that communities care about and love, find the lines blurred between their own identities, the brands they have built, and the power that comes with that. The Ego Eradicator kriyā supports a physical and emotional opening that releases fear, worry and attachment.

The Ego Eradicator kriyā includes kapālabhāti kriyā, the breathing technique described in the previous chapter, which can have calming and positive effects in moments of fear and anxiety. Breaking through narratives of the mind and finding the right path may become available to you after practising this. In a short amount of time, the electromagnetic field surrounding the physical body is energized, the lungs and breathways are opened, the mind is awakened to alertness and, potentially, a person becomes more centred and content.

Practice Break: Ego Eradicator Kriyā

Let us move into the practice.

Take a comfortable seated position. If you are on the floor, it is recommended that you sit in either vajrāsana (diamond pose) or sukhāsana (easy cross-legged position). You can also sit in a chair.

Take the arms up to a 60-degree angle on either side of the body. Keep the elbows straight. The shoulders should be moving down and away from the ears. Do not harden the lower back.

Curl the fingertips onto the pads of the palms at the base of the fingers. Thumbs are stretched back, pointing toward each other.

Close the eyes. Allow the internal gaze to turn toward ājñā chakra – linked to the brow or Third Eye.

Begin kapālabhāti kriyā (see page 95).

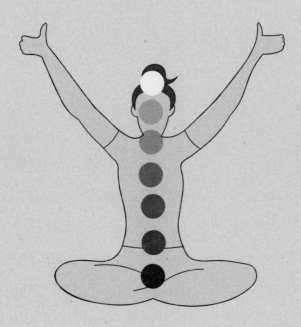

Continue for one to three minutes, depending on your capacity and current practice.

At the end of this time, inhale deeply. Bring the arms overhead so that the thumb tips just about touch. Hold at the top of the breath.

Open the fingers, exhale and release the arms down.

Place the hands on the thighs, palms facing upward, and pause for a few breaths with the eyes still closed.

Let us now turn our attention to integrating these principles into our lives, on and off the mat.

PART IV

SATYA: OUR COLLECTIVE PATHS OF FREEDOM

Satya, truthfulness, is the second yama. Truth or truthfulness is simple and complex at the same time. In yoga and wellness spaces, there is often a lot of talk about speaking one's truth. Sometimes it becomes necessary to ask to what end truth is being spoken. Is it being spoken to convince or persuade others of a particular position? Is it being spoken to establish hierarchy or maintain power dynamics? Is it being spoken out of need, desperation, desire or exasperation? Without ahiṃsā, the principle of nonviolence, there can be no satya. As we continue in our commitment to our practice, we may find that some truth speaking can be delivered and/or land with a degree of violence.

To break those patterns, it can help to be reminded of the difference between truth and Truth, which the teachings of Yoga also address. Each person, with their own point of departure, experiences their own reality wherein their understanding of truth originates. And then there is a Universal Truth that we aspire to tap into through practice. These are not mutually exclusive, but it can be difficult to see through the personal truths to reach the Truth.

Our collective freedom depends on our willingness to acknowledge the differing truths of our fellow human beings, while maintaining that there is no scarcity of Truth. The revolution will be messy, and that's ok.

CHAPTER 9

THE CASE FOR A GLOBAL INDUSTRY CHARTER

Charters have been an instrument of accountability and change across many industries over the last several decades. Charters typically address environmental or social issues that are specific to the industry, relate to current social demands, and/or have the potential to transform the shape of the industry. In science and technology industries, for example, you will find charters that aim to attract more women. In the fashion industry, there are charters to achieve more sustainable practices in order to slow climate change. In the health and wellness industries, there are charters to ensure the scientific rigour of health benefit claims.

This chapter sets out what a charter for the yoga and wellness industry could look like. The charter focuses on cultural appreciation, sustainability, racial and intersectional equity. For such a charter to have an impact, it would need to be a global charter with signatories across different sectors, including but not limited to teachers, studios and gyms, teacher training schools, and online video libraries, as well as companies that produce yoga equipment (including clothes).

The effects of the Covid-19 pandemic have meant that today more people practise at home. Before the pandemic, only 9 per cent of teachers and 40 per cent of students practised yoga online. During the pandemic, the numbers reached 86 per cent of teachers and 91 per cent of students teaching and practising online, respectively. It is too early to know if this trend will continue, but we can assume that yoga has become more accessible through online classes. That means more teachers can make a living outside of the yoga studio, and more people will buy their own equipment. Demand for yoga equipment grew by 154 per cent during the Covid-19 pandemic. The global yoga market size is predicted to grow to $66.2 billion by 2027. There is no better time to act than now.

The Framework

The charter for the yoga and wellness industry would acknowledge and honour the past, present and future Yogins of the Indian subcontinent, who live a life of service to the continuation of the cultural, spiritual and educational practice of Yoga.

The foundation of the charter is comprised of the four core principles of respect, relatedness, repair and reintegration.

Respect: The origins of the wisdom tradition of Yoga lie on the subcontinent of India. It is a living tradition that has been shaped and re-shaped over millennia. We maintain that no one person can own a wisdom tradition. We recognize that modern Yoga was, in part, a response to British colonial rule. We celebrate that Indian sages disseminated their teachings to all parts of the world. We accept that humans are imperfect and such imperfections may influence the teachings, yet the underlying Truth remains intact.

Relatedness: Yoga, as a physical and spiritual practice, lives in all geographies. Practitioners and participants of all backgrounds are connected through Yoga practice to the common ancestry of its origin. Individual actors have the power to cause harm through denying the interconnectedness of individual actions on the collective. We seek to utilize the relatedness of the practice to the benefit of people and the planet.

Repair: Through the hyper-commodification and misappropriation of Yoga as a mere fitness or exercise regime, harm has been caused. The harm to those of South Asian heritage and a Yoga lineage cannot be quantified. The neoliberal pursuits of hyper-commodification and hyper-consumerism have caused immeasurable harm to the planet. We strive to create inclusive processes of repair that acknowledge past or historical injuries with sincerity and humility in order to make amends.

Reintegration: To create an equitable and sustainable future, work is required of all of us. We are charged to work with integrity to become better stewards of the Earth, its land and all living beings. We divest ourselves of systems that were created to serve racial hierarchy. We collectively establish new ways of manufacturing, producing, working and consuming that allow individuals of all backgrounds, bodies and communities to flourish.

There are six key actions to amplify your commitment to a more equitable and sustainable yoga and wellness industry:

1. Educate yourselves about the roots of Yoga.
2. Measure, measure, measure.
3. Embrace courageous conversations.
4. Commit to zero.
5. Embed equity and sustainability into your strategy.
6. Take action that centres the Global Majority.

While the essential elements of these steps are explained below, they will look different for the different actors; for example, teachers versus brands. There is, however, a role for every charter participant or signatory to play in all of these actions. Let's consider each action in turn.

I. Educate Yourselves about the Roots of Yoga

It is not necessary to get a postgraduate degree in Yoga, but it is fundamental to any change process that all participants educate themselves about Yoga's roots. Many of the sacred texts can be downloaded freely, as can translations of them, as they are old enough to be accessed at no cost. A number of scholars have made their publications available to the general public. These articles and essays are useful in providing interpretations and context for ancient texts. Further, it is necessary to understand the effects of British colonial rule on present-day South Asia. In order to decolonize the industry, its actors must first understand what took place during colonial rule and how this still impacts nation states today.

2. Measure, Measure, Measure

In order to establish a baseline and evaluate progress, it is necessary to capture all kinds of data relating to your vision of change. As teachers, for example, you may want to measure who is attending your classes and who is missing. As a studio, you can refer back to chapter 6 for tips on what to measure. All companies and individuals need to measure the impact of their work on the environment.

3. Embrace Courageous Conversations

Courageous conversations are a somewhat trendy practice. When facilitated skilfully, they can lead to real change. Individuals, communities and companies lead courageous conversations to effectively engage in dialogue to transmute deeply rooted assumptions, biases and prejudices about the marginalized and minoritized across any number of social identity categories. These categories should not be treated as siloes, and race must be centred. Such conversations should be facilitated by external partners (e.g., coaches) with expertise in intersectional frameworks and of marginalized identities.

4. Commit to Zero

Organizations must commit to net zero. Net zero refers to balancing the carbon emitted into the atmosphere with the amount of carbon removed from it. Individuals and organizations also commit to zero tolerance for bullying, gaslighting and (online) harassment. Leaders must tackle reports of any form of harassment from both internal and external stakeholders. In organizations, this will mean creating reporting and accountability processes if these do not already exist.

5. Embed Equity and Sustainability into your Strategy

Taking an equity and sustainability lens to your organizational strategy means ensuring that your business is prepared for the future. Hold leaders of your business to account by including equity and sustainability goals as a part of your performance management process. It can be included in variable compensation in organizations where that is applicable. It should also be included in overall performance measures that are reviewed on an annual basis.

6. Take Action that Centres the Global Majority

The Global Majority have endured. Do your part to support a shift from endurance to thriving. After centuries of colonization, exploitation and targeted injustice, the violence persists. It may be less overt or obvious (and sometimes not), but across geographies Indigenous nations and people of African descent still suffer disproportionately across most socio-economic measures. Yet they are also written out of conversations. From campaigns to slow climate change to improving social mobility, centre those who are most negatively impacted by the negligent actions of generations past.

The Process

In order for the charter to be meaningful, signatories would have to be held to account. That means there would need to be a verification and certification process. Signing up to the charter alone would likely not be enough of a distinction or motivation to achieve the type of accelerated transformation that is intended.

At the same time, the yoga and wellness industry is varied and includes everything from solopreneurs to multinational corporations. The verification and certification process must not be overcomplicated or overly expensive, which would disincentivize smaller business owners and sole traders from taking the necessary steps. As a global charter, it could also be too complex to create legal accountability across different markets. These are questions that a governing body would need to consider.

However, there are some key elements to include in any certification process. Products and services alone are not enough to secure certification. A holistic approach to assessing products and services as well as their (positive) impact on people and the planet must be taken. Reporting and transparency guidelines would need to be established to guarantee comparability and replicability across businesses and markets. Finally, a governing body with third-party validation in a not-for-profit structure would be tasked with building trust and value. The governing body must consist of a representative group of people who reflect *all* parts of society.

The Commitment

In acknowledgment of the fact that there is no one way to lead a transformation process and to minimize a hierarchical approach to charter submissions, it is recommended that companies create their own draft of commitments which would then be reviewed by the governing body. The governing body would offer detailed feedback before accepting the submitted commitments or requesting some adjustments. This process creates space for companies to co-create an inclusive process with internal and external stakeholders, who can have a say in what commitments would be meaningful for the communities affected as well as for the planet.

The general format for commitments would include four core commitments that align to the four principles of respect, relatedness, repair and reintegration. These commitments should be bold and ambitious. The four core commitments would be followed by at least six additional statements on how the four core commitments are to be enacted through the use of the six key actions listed on pages 113–14. The minimum six key actions should be explicit in their intentions, rather than using targets. The differentiation of targets and intentions is not merely semantics. Often, targets lead individuals to only look at the end state, or destination, with complete disregard for the process leading to that desired end state. If the focus is on intentions, there is less pressure to reach a target, which means the integrity of the process plays a more central role. The world is constantly in a state of change, so targets might not be the best way to measure progress. The purpose of the charter is not to have individuals and companies take shortcuts in order to appear to be doing the right thing. Instead, the charter is meant to support a process of repair and recalibration, so that we can collectively create an equitable and sustainable future.

JOURNALING PROMPTS

This chapter concludes with journaling prompts instead of a practice. I invite readers to envision a global community committed to equity and sustainability in yoga and wellness. You are invited to dream big. Try to tap into the collective wisdom that there are possibilities beyond what you may be able to conceive or imagine at this time.

» How has Yoga informed who you are today?

» What potential lies within the yoga and wellness industry to positively impact health outcomes (physical, mental, emotional) of people, irrespective of their socio-economic location?

» What becomes possible when the yoga and wellness industry create equitable and inclusive workplaces and practice spaces in which people of all backgrounds can actively participate and bring their full potential?

> » What inner barriers reveal themselves to you when you consider the scope of this work? What underlies these barriers? How can you make them a part of your personal commitment to change?
>
> » What personal commitments aligned with the four core principles of respect, relatedness, repair and reintegration are you willing to make today?

CHAPTER 10

OFF THE MAT: LIVING THESE PRINCIPLES BEYOND A STUDIO ENVIRONMENT

For those of you who are among the TL;DR persuasion, this chapter is for you. Throughout this book, I have offered different frameworks to support your building your own capacity to make good decisions in critical moments. This chapter is a bit more hands-on, offering examples across different roles. I would really encourage you to read previous chapters relating to your work in the yoga and wellness industry, whether that be as a teacher, studio owner, brand manager or otherwise. At the same time, I recognize that the examples offered in this chapter can help to make even more tangible some of the nuances of previous chapters.

Yoga and Wellness Practitioners

Don't be lazy.

Don't ignore the lack of diversity you see in wellness spaces. Do ask space holders what their equity and inclusion strategy is. The ask doesn't have to be public or loud. It just needs to be sincere. Indicate to the places you patronize that you care about these things and that you are paying attention. Let them know that there will be consequences for their inaction.

Don't stick to the familiar. Do visit classes from different teachers. We all develop some form of attachment to the teachers whose styles resonate with us. That's human. We now have the opportunity, more than ever, to venture out and to learn from teachers who are, for example, from and based in South Asia. Increasing numbers of teachers provide virtual offerings due to the pandemic. It may feel unfamiliar and thus uncomfortable. But do it anyway. And don't compare your experiences. Simply feel confident that you can find teachers you love all across the world, and some of them should be in South Asia.

Don't act like equity in the yoga and wellness industry is too big for you to influence. Do feel a sense of responsibility to play your part. We each have a part to play. You've likely heard the African proverb about the mosquito in the room, or experienced an actual mosquito in your bedroom in the middle of the night. If we as individuals don't believe that we can be a part of the change, why should anyone make the first step? No matter how insignificant you think your contribution may be, rest assured that – whether positive or negative – your action can ripple through the collective.

Don't take things personally. If you make a mistake and someone calls you on it, that's ok. It's a learning opportunity. The only thing that makes it not ok is the inner narrative that believes mistakes make you a bad person. They do not. The mistake isn't nearly as important as what you choose to do next. Choose to do the work so that you can do better.

DO	DON'T
Do ask space holders what their equity and inclusion strategy is.	Don't ignore the lack of diversity you see in wellness spaces.
Do visit classes from different teachers.	Don't stick to the familiar.
Do feel a sense of responsibility.	Don't act like it's not your problem.
Do the work to do better.	Don't take it personally.

Teachers/Yoga Influencers

Don't speak *for.*

If you are racialized as white, do not speak on behalf of teachers who identify as Black, Indigenous or as people of colour. Instead, make referrals and pass on such offers to BIPOC teachers who can then speak for themselves.

If you are racialized as white, it is not your place to speak on the matter of cultural appropriation. Instead, you can point to BIPOC teachers, who have already been talking and writing on the subject.

If you are racialized as white, don't call yourself antiracist. Instead, do the work, read the books, and have conversations among your white peers about your internalized racism, which shows up as internalized white supremacy. If you are a non-Black person of colour, you will also need to commit to doing work around anti-Black racism, how it may have been internalized and how it shows up in your communities. BIPOC folks of non-South Asian heritage need to investigate to what extent they are replicating bad behaviours of dominant culture in yoga spaces. Moreover, we all have work to do to become better allies, especially in environments where people with different social identities have no representation. People who identify as heterosexual must show up for their LGBTQ+ peers. Cis folks need to do work to better understand the existential risks trans- and non-binary folks face in everyday circumstances. Non-disabled people need to deepen their understanding for the myriad ways that people with visible and invisible disabilities are prevented from fully participating in yoga and wellness spaces. Don't forget: your default for these different identities may be white. Do the research to understand the specific needs and challenges of BIPOC folks with multiple marginalized identities.

Irrespective of your racialization, never become complacent. Don't get a seat at the table and find yourself satisfied. BIPOC folks feel a lot of pressure when they are in the room alone.[20] White people treat them as if they are speaking on behalf of an entire community (newsflash – impossible). They may be struggling with feelings of internalized racism that indicate they "deserve" to be there or not (no bootstrap rhetoric, please), or they are faced with the critical judgement of nepotism and/or insatiability if they argue to bring more of the underrepresented into the room (notice how this is only an issue for minoritized folks, not for dominant culture). Bring them anyway.

DO	DON'T
Do pass speaking engagements and other offers on to teachers who identify as Black, Indigenous, and people of colour (BIPOC).	If you are racialized as white, don't speak on behalf of BIPOC teachers.
Do point to BIPOC teachers who are talking and writing about cultural appropriation.	If you are racialized as white, don't talk about cultural appropriation.
Do the work to do better.	Don't proclaim to be antiracist or an ally.
Do bring other people with underrepresented identities to the table.	Don't get in the room and be happy to stay there alone.

Teacher Trainers

Don't get it twisted.

Don't perpetuate the system that centres white faculty as experts. This is directed at people of all races and ethnicities. Internalized racism/white supremacy shows up in this way. There is a credibility that is automatically lent to white teachers that is hard-earned among BIPOC teachers. Do prioritize learning from and uplifting BIPOC yoga and wellness teachers.

There is no need to diminish the statement with additions such as "BIPOC yoga and wellness teachers who are equally as qualified". This too is an expression of internalized racism.

Don't accept colonized credentialing pathways. If we look to the end of the 19th and beginning of the 20th centuries, Indian master teachers were not offering accreditation for teacher trainings. The pathway was a shared journey. Of course, there are flaws in the master–student relationship, as it leaves students vulnerable to the (good) will of the master. One of its greatest strengths, however, has been completely removed from the western credentialing pathway: the focus on the process rather than the end goal. This means that the experience of someone who grew up practising Yoga is rendered irrelevant, but a person who was certified while on a month-long holiday in an exotic location, can be called qualified. In comparable fields of exercise, fitness, therapeutics and healing, it is unheard of to certify someone as a teacher (or leader) after just 27 days.

Don't replicate poor pedagogy. Pedagogy is defined as the theory and practice of learning. As bell hooks explains, "Teachers must be aware of themselves as practitioners and as human beings if they wish to teach students in a non-threatening, anti-discriminatory way. Self-actualization should be the goal of the teacher as well as the students."[21] Don't think that the students have little to nothing to offer. Develop a teaching practice that allows your trainees to co-create the space with you. This will support their professional development as teachers and provide a living example of how they can create inclusive spaces with their future students.

Don't fall into the trap of needing to know everything and having all the answers in the role of the teacher. If you are being challenged by trainees, then use it as a learning opportunity. If you're being challenged by peers, then ask them for their insights and listen to what they have to say. If you're feeling unsettled by this book, know there are many books that can fill the gaps in your knowledge which may have been revealed in your time here. Let go of the resistance and do the work to do better.

DO	DON'T
Do learn from and uplift BIPOC yoga and wellness teachers.	Don't perpetuate the system that maintains all white faculty as the experts.
Do enter into dialogue with governing bodies to demand change.	Don't accept colonized credentialing pathways.
Do co-create spaces with trainees.	Don't replicate poor pedagogy.
Do the work to do better.	Don't believe you have all the answers.

Yoga and Wellness Brands

Don't believe the hype.

Don't tokenize marginalized talent. And don't believe that it's ok to tokenize talent because "they went along with it". At the end of the day, we all have to make our choices, and if it is between work or no work, exposure or no exposure, most folks will choose the work or unpaid exposure. That's nothing to feel great about as a brand. Instead, devote time to building, nurturing and maintaining meaningful relationships with underrepresented community members. For example, don't just use paid partnerships with specific influencers to reach untapped audiences if you have nothing to offer that audience. Enter into dialogue with that audience. Understand what that audience cares about. Develop a relationship. Don't just demand their attention.

Don't pinch pennies. After the social justice protests of 2020, companies showed the world how much money is available to spend on racial equity and social justice when there's energy behind it. We will no longer believe that there is no budget available for the welfare of underrepresented stakeholders. Do invest in learning experiences, internally as well as externally. Take stakeholders on the (un-)learning journey with you.

Don't think your brand is too big to fail. As discussed in chapter 8, the relationship between consumers and brands has changed. Brands have felt the consequences of playing on Team Bad Decisions. Socially conscious consumers are happy to put their money where their mouth is. They will delete an app that is showing poor judgement in a critical moment. Influencers will strike or boycott when they recognize that they are being neglected, underserved and underpaid. Leverage the power of your brand for social good. Use your brand to spread messages of equity, sustainability and collective empowerment. The best way to spread that message is by overhauling your internal practices to better reflect the change you want to see in the world.

Don't cut corners. It is not enough to take some pretty pictures and put it on your platform. Consumers will notice, and they will call you out. This work doesn't begin in the marketing and communications teams. Instead, demand that the board, the executive committee and other senior leaders are held to account for the decisions that they make. More senior executives must recognize that they make better decisions for the brand and for themselves when they do the work.

DO	DON'T
Do devote time to building and maintaining meaningful relationships with underrepresented community members.	Don't tokenize marginalized talent.
Do invest in learning experiences.	Don't pinch pennies.
Do leverage your brand power for good.	Don't think your brand is too big to fail.
Do the work to do better.	Don't cut corners.

Can You See the Change?

Often, people on panels broadly discussing diversity, equity and inclusion use some version of the saying "be the change you want to see". Therein lies an important question, though. Can people actually see the change? There are many reasons that they may not see the change. You don't know what you don't know, which makes it slightly difficult to know all that needs changing. Harder still can be confronting the internal blocks that don't allow you to dive into the expansiveness of unknown possibilities.

Building on the last chapter's journaling prompts, you are now invited into a guided visualization to support you in giving yourself the freedom to dream, and to dream big. To envision the things that may not seem possible today. To feel the things that are greater than what is known to us today. This may seem unrealistic, and it should. For those of us with minoritized identities, it's hard to imagine a world in which we are completely free. It can be an important first step to imagine what that kind of freedom even feels like.

Practice Break: Visualization

Let's move into practice. It could be useful to practise in groups so that one person reads the instructions in real time. Alternatively, you can record yourself saying the text and listen back to it. This guided visualization can be drawn out for as long as you like or shortened to five minutes. It's up to you.

Find a quiet place to sit or lie down. Turn your phone on to "do not disturb". Know that this is your time to relax and come into stillness. Notice if you need anything before completely settling down. Take whatever you may need; for example, a blanket or socks to keep yourself warm. Ensure that you will be able to stay in your chosen position for the next several minutes.

Bring your awareness to rest on your breath, without trying to control its depth or rhythm. If your breath is not available to you at this time, rest your awareness at the area just below your navel.

Continue to observe your breath or the sensations below the navel. As thoughts arise, observe the nature of your thoughts, and then bring your attention back to your anchor (either your breath or the area just below the navel). As your body relaxes more and more, you can allow the mind to relax further as you focus on the guided imagery, which begins now . . .

Take some time to see and honour every place you have been up until now. Hold gratitude in your heart for all of your life's twists and turns. Celebrate the gift that you are still here, still learning.

Take a few more intentional, deeper breaths before continuing on this journey.

Tune in to the sensory experience of the body, including the sounds around you.

Where do you experience discrimination in your body? Where are you holding experiences of alienation in your body? Can you tune in to these parts of the body without replaying the events in your mind?

What would it feel like to let go of some of that holding? Can you release some of it now, even just by a tiny amount?

Take a few more intentional, deeper breaths before continuing on this journey.

Observe the nature of the thoughts arising in this moment. Notice how the nature of your thoughts connects with different parts of your body. What would it feel like in your body to be free of judging thoughts? What would it feel like in your body to be free of thoughts of having to prove yourself, or to be deserving of validation?

As you release some of the holding and feel into the freedom of non-judgement, bring to mind someone you care about. Someone with whom your relationship is in good, uncomplicated standing. Allow them to be present before you. How does this release affect how you engage with them? What feels different in your body?

Call before you more members of your community. Now that you're a little bit freer, what does it feel like to be in relationship with them?

Take a few more intentional, deeper breaths.

Observe what has shifted in your body. Allow your awareness to flow from the feet to the head and back down again. What do you notice?

What does just a bit more freedom feel like in your body?

Allow your breath to deepen.

When you are ready, you can begin to gently reawaken your body and mind.

Slowly return to the presence of the space you are currently inhabiting.

Feel your muscles reawakening as you take note of your surroundings.

You may want to stretch, feeling into the body more as you fully awaken.

CHAPTER 11

THE BALANCE OF SELF-ENQUIRY AND ACTIONABLE STRATEGIES

In this book, I have tried to balance a few aims: providing guidance on how to approach taking action; rooting all actions in Yoga, the wisdom tradition; and leaving space for the reader's own process. The book will not have answered all readers' questions. No book can claim that. It focuses primarily on creating a framework for change for the primary actors in the yoga and wellness industry. The journaling prompts are an opportunity for readers to reflect on the content of the book, as well as personal experiences that connect to that content. The practices at the end of the chapters are intended to support readers in allowing whatever comes up to emerge. To leave room for a response rather than to fall into old reactive patterns. This, in turn, supports us in responding more wisely to social and racial injustice.

Once you have started on this path, there is no turning back. It becomes impossible to unsee what has been revealed to you. As we deepen our practice by connecting it more palpably to the things taking place in the world around us, it becomes harder to tune the world out or remain wholly invested in previous assumptions and biases. That can feel uncomfortable. As this book repeatedly states, there is no certainty, no singular right way to journey on this path. That can feel uncomfortable. There is nowhere to turn for all the right answers, and there is no guarantee of no longer making mistakes or getting things right, even with the greatest of intentions. That definitely feels uncomfortable.

Yogins Just Wanna Have Fun

By now, some readers might be truly tired of hearing about staying with or allowing their discomfort. I get it. There are moments where social media bombards us with the realities of the precarious nature of inhabiting a marginalized body in this world. In these moments, the majority of us share a sense of urgency to make changes. But, eventually, that sense of urgency subsides, and we just want to go back to our lives. For some that means feeling full of contentment after (physical or posture) practice. Things feel easier. Sure, you might donate to a cause, which makes you feel better, but you're not faced with precarity. It does not come up in your inner circles, and you're able to lead the lifestyle you've chosen for yourself.

Again, others may be very familiar with the feeling of a precarious life. Whether it be due to income or job insecurity, or some other issue that challenges your daily existence, you know what it means to be one illness or injury or late notice away from chaos. You may be irked by feeling that you are being asked to see yourself as privileged and in need of making some changes too. You would prefer that there is some acknowledgment and recognition of your own struggles. Yoga helps you feel better about and manage life's curveballs, and there is no reason you should have to change that.

There are surely some readers who feel like the book doesn't go far enough, doesn't demand nearly enough of the major industry players such as brands. It may read as though multinationals are being treated with equal tenderness and patience as individual actors with only minimal power. There's certainly nothing radical about that, amirite?

Even though you might have assumptions, notice that I did not explicitly add any protected social identity categories to the above descriptions. That's on purpose. I'll leave you to reflect on your assumptions and how they informed your reaction to the scenarios. More importantly is, perhaps, the universality of aversion. Aversion shows up in multiple ways, more than the previous paragraphs illustrated. But aversion, or resistance, is always a good indication of themes that require more attention.

Fear It and Do It Anyway

One common concern that arises in my trainings, most often from participants who are racialized as white, is a fear of saying something wrong. But it's not just that. The fear is about *inadvertently* saying the "wrong thing" that *unintentionally* causes harm or injury, or – perhaps even worse – incriminates you as ignorant, offensive or racist. Unfortunately, most people who raise this reduce their concern to language. This is not a mere matter of word choice. Word choice points to an underlying frame of reference of the speaker. Language is one window into recognizing perspective. Yet language is rapidly adapting to our new understandings of social justice issues. If you fear using the wrong words, then you are likely missing the greater learning opportunity. And that dead angle (or lack of mindfulness) shows up in your choice of speech.

Similarly, a concern for one's actions being received as inauthentic comes up often. What underlines these concerns is the understanding of "self". The concerns convey a deeper desire to uphold one's image of oneself than to dig into the work. As we grow older, the tendency is to become more self-conscious. Indeed, it is one function of the collective or community. There is a sometimes subtle and sometimes overt punishment and reward system that teaches us from an early age what behaviour is acceptable and what is not. It informs the self-image that we create of ourselves. It is likely a safe bet that for the majority of people, that self-image does not include cultural appropriator, oppressor or racist. In today's social media context in which the word "racist" is used as a standalone (versus for example racist policies, racist actions, etc.), people are often concerned with being cancelled for reasons beyond their intentions.

I urge you to move through the fear. You must do the work, and you must maintain your practice. Is there another example of something you have learned where your fear of getting it wrong proved greater than your aspiration to do better? Playing an instrument, riding a bicycle, learning āsana? What is different here? Fear of getting things wrong is not reason enough to not do the work, or to only do enough to keep up appearances. Have you ever experienced a student who desperately wanted to learn (or *conquer*) an āsana? They come to class with the expectation that you can teach them how to get into the posture. They apply force. And they become frustrated when it doesn't work on the first couple of tries. Then, paths part. Some students become so frustrated that they stop coming to your class altogether. Others continue to practise other postures – at home and in your class. Then one day, perhaps six months later, you're teaching the posture again, and the student moves into it with ease. They may not hold the posture for long, but they get a glimpse of what it feels like to be in the posture, albeit briefly. They now know what they were missing and what still needs work. It's similar. The shift cannot be taught, and it doesn't come with force. It comes with consistent practice over an extended period of time. And even when you get it, it's not necessarily pretty.

Readers must not go away from this book and claim they still have so much to learn that they are not yet prepared to take immediate action. The smallest well-informed actions will pave the way for lasting change. Equally, I ask that readers do not put this book down feeling accomplished, as if the work is now done. The work is never done. See that as a liberating truth. There is nowhere you have to get to, nowhere you need to be by a given time and date. This book is a starting point or continuation. Readers start where they are with what they have. The work continues over the course of our entire lives. At times, it will be incredibly challenging, and yet it is always worth doing to create systems and spaces that benefit all.

Action, Action, We Want Action

Over the course of the book, I have provided actions that different actors can take. In the previous chapter, you can find a short list of some immediate actions that you can take on pages 119–25, depending on your role in the yoga and wellness industry. In the following, I reiterate some of the overarching themes:

- Readers racialized as white are asked to take these conversations forward to friends, families and their communities. The work is something that should be done in relationship with other folks. In relationship it becomes possible to learn, to figure things out, and to build resilience.

- The practice is having conversations that call people in through compassionate yet candid communication. The conversations don't have to end in agreement. But you do have to seek to hold conversations that make it possible for the listeners to receive your message as you intended. It doesn't mean they will get it or agree with it. But no one benefits from conversations where everyone is talking (or defending), and no one is listening. Seeds are ultimately planted in such moments, and you have to be good with the fact that you may never see them bloom.

- While this book focuses on Yoga, there is transferable knowledge for spaces and industries beyond yoga and wellness. You cannot fully show up on the mat if you are not showing up for social justice and racial equity off it.

This book is just the beginning.

Closing Practice: Samavṛtti Prāṇāyāma

Samavṛtti prāṇāyāma, equal or box breathing, is a breath technique to come back to any time you are feeling stressed, anxious or overwhelmed. It is referred to as box or equal breathing because the breath is taken in equal parts using a count of four. A box, or square, has four sides of equal lengths. If, at any time, you become stressed or feel extremely unsettled, discontinue the retention of the breath. Open your eyes. Bring your awareness to an anchor point; for example, your connection to the Earth.

Let us move into the practice. You can practise this any time of day, or in any moment you feel your blood pressure rising or stressed. It is best practised alone and at your own rhythm.

Come, with intention, into a comfortable seated position. You can also practise standing. Lying down is less optimal. If seated, place your hands in your lap – one on top of the other. Alternatively, you can place the hands on the thighs – palms up for opening or palms down for grounding. If standing, allow the hands to relax by either side, turning the palms to face forward.

Exhale to empty the breath from the lungs.

Inhale through the nose to a count of four. Don't worry about how long a count of four is. Just try to keep the same rhythm for your count throughout.

Pause at the top of the breath for a count of four. Hold the breath in.

Exhale through the nose for a count of four. (You can also inhale and exhale through the mouth if the nose is stuffy.)

Pause at the bottom of the breath for a count of four. Hold the breath out.

Repeat steps three through six for three to four rounds. As you build in your practice, you can repeat for several rounds and/or you can increase your count to six or eight.

Once you finish, simply allow the breath to flow, without retention, at its own rhythm.

NOTES

1   The word "Yoga" is capitalized when referring to its origins, the wisdom tradition, etc., while lower case is used for the secular practice in, for example, western yoga classes. I understand that this may not be a perfect separation, as not all classes should be treated as the same. However, this is the most consistent way to differentiate between these approaches and make it easier for the reader to perceive the differences between the two.

2   It should be noted that the mention of God is another difference between the Sāṅkhya and the Yoga doctrines. Sāṅkhya could be considered atheistic in nature as, in its classical form, it speaks of the supremacy of spirit, but there is no God. And the understanding of God here differs from the God of the Upaniṣads in that God, in this instance, is not all-encompassing.

3   *Bhagavadgītā*, translated from the Sanskrit by Swami Nikhilananda in 1944 and published by Ramakrishna-Vivekananda Center, New York City, reprint 2004.

4   I acknowledge that people of colour as well as Black and Indigenous people are disproportionately imprisoned. This project does not address the root problem. It does, however, serve these communities in their current circumstances which is reported as being received as supportive by the people taking part.

5   You can read more on this in Elliott Goldberg's *The Path of Modern Yoga: The History of an Embodied Spiritual Practice*, Inner Traditions, Rochester, 2016.

6   As quoted in *Autobiography of a Yogi* by Paramhansa Yogananda, published by Crystal Clarity Publishers, Nevada City, 1995, p. 144.

Reprint of the 1946 first edition published by The Philosophical Library, New York City.

7   The Yoga Alliance website is: https://www.yogaalliance.org/. (These details were last updated on 29 June 2020.)

8   See, for example, the 2019 Netflix documentary *Bikram: Yogi, Guru, Predator*, directed by Eva Orner.

9   I reject the notion that any modern-day western practitioner can "found" Yoga. They can adapt what is an ancient practice to their personal desires and needs. Then the question presents itself if that can still even be called Yoga. In any case, it cannot be a claim to have founded Yoga, irrespective of the names they place before the word Yoga.

10   See, for example, Michelle Goldberg, "A Workplace, an Ashram, or a Cult? Inside the sexual harassment lawsuit against Jivamukti Yoga", The Slate Group, 5 April 2016. Available at: https://slate.com/human-interest/2016/04/jivamukti-sexual-harassment-lawsuit-says-the-yoga-studio-is-a-cult.html; Sarah Herrington, "Yoga Teachers Need a Code of Ethics", *New York Times*, 7 June 2017, and Matthew Remski, "Silence and Silencing at Jivamukti Yoga and Beyond", Decolonizing Yoga, 1 June 2016. Available at: http://decolonizingyoga.com/silence-silencing-jivamukti-yoga-beyond/.

11   Yoga Alliance International is India's first international yoga alliance. It is not affiliated with US-based Yoga Alliance.

12   This statement was delivered in Morrison's commencement speech to the graduating class of 1979 at Barnard College.

13   Kimberlé Crenshaw, "Why Intersectionality Can't Wait", *Washington Post*, 24 September 2015. Available at https://www.washingtonpost.com/news/in-theory/wp/2015/09/24/why-intersectionality-cant-wait/

14   See Robin Ely and David A. Thomas, "Getting Serious About Diversity: Enough Already with the Business Case", *Harvard Business Review*, 98, no. 6 (November–December 2020).

15   It is up to you which version of the threat question you seek to answer. It may also be interesting to allow different groups to evaluate one of the two questions. Groups that are especially resistant to this work may be better served in answering the latter question.

16   The interview was conducted by Jonelle Lewis for the purpose of this book in December 2021. Deep gratitude to Leanne Adu for

transcribing the interview. (Minor edits have been made to ensure flow and understanding of the conversation.)

17   Bedford–Stuyvesant, colloquially known as Bed–Stuy, is a neighbourhood in the northern section of the New York City borough of Brooklyn.

18   I use the term "safe enough" here to acknowledge that it is not possible for public spaces to be "safe" spaces. Public spaces should, however, strive to be safe enough for people to enter without fear of great or enduring harm.

19   As a Diploma Course Tutor, a teacher is contracted by the BWY Training unit to deliver the Diploma course.

20   This example works for (white) women too.

21   b. hooks, *Teaching to Transgress: Education as the Practice of Freedom*, Routledge, New York, 1994.

GLOSSARY

BIPOC: Black, Indigenous, People of Colour – a term widely used in North America.

Cis(gender): A term for people whose gender identity matches their designated sex at birth.

Diversity: The addition of people of different backgrounds (across a myriad of social categories) in a group, team or organization.

Dominant culture: A cultural practice whose language, faith or spiritual traditions, values and customs are taken as the norm in a political or societal entity in which several cultures coexist.

Equity: The treatment of people with unique needs as equal.

Guṇa: A quality, attribute or property of nature. There are three complementary forces: *tamas* (inertia, lethargy), *rajas* (passion, vibrancy) and *sattva* (luminosity, purity).

Imperialism: A policy or ideology of extending or imposing power, authority, or influence over sovereign lands, territories, or nations.

Inclusion: A policy or practice of including and accommodating people who have historically been excluded into the default, general or normed population.

Marginalize: An act, policy or practice of disempowering a person or group to such an extent that they cannot fully participate in society.

Minoritize: An act, policy or practice of subjecting a person or group to differential and disadvantageous treatment that constrains their participation in a team, organization or society at large.

Neoliberalism: A term to describe free-market capitalism, which as an ideology positions freedom as an inherent social value that sees the role of the state minimized or reduced.

Oppression: Defined by the *Merriam-Webster Dictionary* as an unjust or cruel exercise of authority or power.

Patriarchy: A social system or ideology that affords men primary power in legal affairs, social freedoms, moral authority and political leadership.

Prakṛti: The original source of the material world, which consists of the three guṇas.

Racialization (or ethnicization): The socio-political act of ascribing racial (or ethnic) identities to a person or group to enable or further oppression.

Sāṅkhya: An Indian philosophy, or school of thought, consisting of a system of 25 true principles to liberate the soul.

Somatics: A field within bodywork which emphasizes the internal perception of the body (soma) as a means to transform and heal.

Spiritual bypassing: The act of using spiritual ideas to escape or avoid interpersonal conflict, psychological wounds, and socio-political issues.

Upaniṣads: Late Vedic texts, written in Sanskrit, commonly referred to as Vedānta. They are the most recent part of the Vedas.

Vedas: A body of sacred texts or scriptures originating on the ancient Indian subcontinent.

White supremacy: A belief system that white or white-presenting people are inherently superior to other races and should therefore dominate and oppress them.

Yoga: A spiritual practice originating on the ancient Indian subcontinent that includes physical and mental disciplines with the aim of stilling the mind and eventually liberating one's soul from repeated suffering.

FURTHER READING

Akala, *Natives: Race and Class in the Ruins of Empire*, Hodder & Stoughton, London, 2018

Barkataki, S., *Embrace Yoga's Roots: Courageous Ways to Deepen Your Yoga Practice*, Ignite Yoga and Wellness Institute, Orlando, 2020

Bhopal, K., *White Privilege: The Myth of a Post-Racial Society*, Policy Press, Bristol, 2018

Eberhardt, J.L., *Biased: The New Science of Race and Inequality*, William Heinemann, London, 2019

Eddo-Lodge, R., *Why I'm No Longer Talking to White People About Race*, Bloomsbury Circus, London, 2017

Emejulu, A. & Sobande, F. (eds), *To Exist is to Resist: Black Feminism in Europe*, Pluto Press, London, 2019

Goldberg, E., *The Path of Modern Yoga: The History of an Embodied Spiritual Practice*, Inner Traditions, Rochester, 2016

Hannah-Jones, N., et al (eds), *The 1619 Project: A New American Origin Story*, Penguin Random House, New York, 2021

Hiriyanna, M., *The Essentials of Indian Philosophy*, Motilal Banarsidass Publishers, Delhi, 2008

hooks, b., *Teaching to Transgress: Education as the Practice of Freedom*, Routledge, Oxon, 1994

hooks, b., *Teaching Community: A Pedagogy of Hope*, Routledge, Oxon, 2003

hooks, b., *Teaching Critical Thinking: Practical Wisdom*, Routledge, Oxon, 2010

Johnson, M.C., *Skill in Action: Radicalizing Your Yoga Practice to Create a Just World*, Shambhala Publications, Boulder, 2021

Kendi, I.X., *How to be an Antiracist*, The Bodley Head, London, 2019

King, R, *Mindful of Race: Transforming Racism from the Inside Out*, Sounds True, Boulder, 2018

Menakem, R., *My Grandmother's Hands: Racialized Trauma and the Pathway to Mending Our Hearts and Bodies*, Central Recovery Press, Las Vegas, 2017

Olusoga, D., *Black and British: A Forgotten History*, Pan Macmillan, 2016

Parker, G., *Restorative Yoga for Ethnic and Race-Based Stress and Trauma*, Jessica Kingsley Publishers, London, 2020

Saad, L.F., *Me and White Supremacy: How to Recognise Your Privilege, Combat Racism and Change the World*, Quercus Editions, London, 2020

williams, a. K. et al, *Radical Dharma: Talking Race, Love, and Liberation*, North Atlantic Books, Berkeley, 2016

Yogananda, P., *Autobiography of a Yogi*, Crystal Clarity Publishers, Nevada City, 1995

INDEX

Note: page numbers in **bold** refer to illustrations.
Page numbers in *italics* refer to information contained in tables.

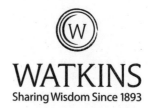

WATKINS

Sharing Wisdom Since 1893

The story of Watkins began in 1893, when scholar of esotericism John Watkins founded our bookshop, inspired by the lament of his friend and teacher Madame Blavatsky that there was nowhere in London to buy books on mysticism, occultism or metaphysics. That moment marked the birth of Watkins, soon to become the publisher of many of the leading lights of spiritual literature, including Carl Jung, Rudolf Steiner, Alice Bailey and Chögyam Trungpa.

Today, the passion at Watkins Publishing for vigorous questioning is still resolute. Our stimulating and groundbreaking list ranges from ancient traditions and complementary medicine to the latest ideas about personal development, holistic wellbeing and consciousness exploration. We remain at the cutting edge, committed to publishing books that change lives.

DISCOVER MORE AT:
www.watkinspublishing.com

Read our blog   Watch and listen to   Sign up to
our authors in action   our mailing list

We celebrate conscious, passionate, wise and happy living.
Be part of that community by visiting

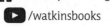 /watkinspublishing   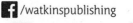 @watkinswisdom
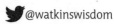 /watkinsbooks   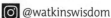 @watkinswisdom